TYPE-2 DIABETES FOOD LIST GUIDE

Empower Your Health with Diabetes-Friendly Foods: A Comprehensive Food List Guide to Optimizing Nutrition and Healthy Diabetic Lifestyle.

Vennesa A Joseph

TABLE OF CONTENTS

CHAPTER 1

INTRODUCTION

1.1 Understanding Type-2 Diabetes

Type-2 diabetes is a chronic metabolic disorder characterized by insulin resistance and inadequate insulin production. To comprehend this condition fully, it's crucial to delve into the intricate mechanisms that regulate blood sugar levels and the factors contributing to its onset.

At its core, diabetes involves the hormone insulin, which plays a pivotal role in glucose metabolism. In individuals with type-2 diabetes, cells become resistant to insulin's effects, impeding the efficient uptake of glucose from the bloodstream. This resistance leads to elevated blood sugar levels, causing various health complications.

Genetic predisposition, sedentary lifestyle, obesity, and poor dietary choices contribute significantly to the development of type-2 diabetes. Understanding this condition's risk factors and early signs is paramount for timely intervention and effective management.

The complex interplay of genetic and environmental factors underscores the importance of a holistic understanding of type-2 diabetes. Genetic predisposition may increase susceptibility, but lifestyle factors often serve as triggers. As we explore the intricate web of causation, it becomes evident that a multifaceted approach to management is essential.

Furthermore, understanding the impact of type-2 diabetes on the body is crucial. Elevated blood sugar levels can lead to complications affecting the heart, kidneys, eyes, and nervous system. Through this understanding, individuals can appreciate the significance of proactive management and lifestyle modifications in preventing these complications.

1.2 Importance of Diet in Managing Diabetes

Diet plays a pivotal role in managing type-2 diabetes. Our food choices directly influence blood sugar levels, making dietary modifications an integral aspect of diabetes management. A balanced and mindful approach to nutrition can positively impact insulin sensitivity and promote overall well-being.

Carbohydrates, in particular, have a profound impact on blood sugar levels. Understanding the distinction between simple and complex carbohydrates empowers individuals to make informed dietary choices.

Incorporating whole grains, legumes, and fibrous vegetables can provide sustained energy without causing rapid spikes in blood sugar.

The role of proteins and fats in diabetes management should not be overlooked. Proteins contribute to satiety and muscle maintenance, while healthy fats play a crucial role in cardiovascular health. Striking the right balance among these macronutrients is essential for a well-rounded and diabetes-friendly diet.

Meal timing and portion control are equally critical. Spreading meals throughout the day and avoiding large, infrequent meals can help regulate blood sugar levels. This approach prevents excessive strain on the pancreas and promotes more stable insulin levels.

Furthermore, the significance of glycemic index (GI) in food choices cannot be overstated. Foods with a high GI can cause rapid spikes in blood sugar, while low-GI foods release glucose more gradually. A diet comprising predominantly low-GI foods can contribute to better blood sugar control.

Dietary choices also influence weight management, a crucial aspect of type-2 diabetes management. Excess body weight, especially around the abdominal region, is closely linked to insulin resistance. Adopting a balanced and calorie-conscious diet can contribute to weight loss and improved insulin sensitivity.

In the context of managing diabetes through diet, individualization is key. Each person's response to different foods varies, highlighting the importance of personalized dietary plans. Monitoring blood sugar levels and observing how the body reacts to different foods enable individuals to tailor their diet to meet their specific needs.

CHAPTER 2

BASICS OF TYPE-2 DIABETES

2.1 Causes and Risk Factors

Understanding the causes and risk factors of type-2 diabetes is crucial for both prevention and effective management. This multifaceted condition is influenced by a combination of genetic, lifestyle, and environmental factors, each playing a unique role in its development.

Genetic Factors:

Genetics can significantly contribute to an individual's susceptibility to type-2 diabetes. Family history often serves as a precursor, highlighting the hereditary nature of the condition. Specific genetic variations can affect insulin production, glucose metabolism, and overall pancreatic function. While genetic predisposition does not guarantee the development of diabetes, it increases the risk, necessitating heightened awareness and preventive measures for individuals with a family history.

Lifestyle Choices:

One of the most influential factors in the onset of type-2 diabetes is lifestyle. Sedentary habits and poor dietary choices, often leading to obesity, contribute significantly to insulin resistance. The modern sedentary lifestyle, characterized by prolonged periods of sitting and minimal physical activity, is closely linked to the rising prevalence of type-2 diabetes. Adopting a more active lifestyle, coupled with mindful dietary habits, can mitigate these risk factors.

Obesity and Body Composition:

Excess body weight, especially abdominal obesity, is a major risk factor for type-2 diabetes. Adipose tissue, particularly around the abdominal area, is metabolically active and can release substances that interfere with insulin function. Understanding the connection between body composition and diabetes risk emphasizes the importance of weight management in diabetes prevention. Achieving and maintaining a healthy weight through a combination of diet and exercise is a cornerstone in reducing the risk of type-2 diabetes.

Age and Ethnicity:

Age and ethnicity also play a role in diabetes risk. While it can occur at any age, the risk increases significantly with age, especially after the age of 45. Certain ethnic groups, such as African Americans, Hispanic/Latino Americans, Native Americans, and Asian Americans, are more prone to developing type-2 diabetes. The reasons for these disparities are complex, involving genetic and environmental factors unique to each population.

Gestational Diabetes:

Women who have experienced gestational diabetes during pregnancy are at an increased risk of developing type-2 diabetes later in life. Gestational diabetes is a temporary condition that affects blood sugar levels during pregnancy. However, it serves as an early warning sign, highlighting the need for continued monitoring and preventive measures post-pregnancy.

Insulin Resistance and Impaired Glucose Tolerance:

Insulin resistance, a key feature of type-2 diabetes, occurs when cells fail to respond adequately to insulin. This condition often precedes the onset of diabetes and can be influenced by genetic factors, obesity, and sedentary lifestyle. Impaired glucose tolerance, another precursor to diabetes, involves higher-than-normal blood sugar levels but not yet in the diabetic range. Understanding these early indicators allows for interventions that can potentially prevent the progression to full-blown diabetes.

2.2 Symptoms and Diagnosis

Recognizing the symptoms of type-2 diabetes is crucial for early diagnosis and effective management. Often, the condition develops gradually, and symptoms may be subtle or overlooked. Understanding the signs and seeking timely medical attention can significantly impact the course of the disease.

Common Symptoms:

The symptoms of type-2 diabetes can vary, and not everyone may experience the same signs. Common indicators include increased thirst and hunger, frequent urination, unexplained weight loss, fatigue, and blurred vision. These symptoms arise as a result of elevated blood sugar levels and the body's attempt to compensate for insulin resistance.

Fatigue and Increased Hunger:

The body's inability to efficiently utilize glucose for energy can lead to persistent fatigue. Despite increased hunger, individuals may experience weight loss due to the breakdown of muscle and fat for energy. These paradoxical symptoms often prompt medical attention and investigations into blood sugar levels.

Frequent Urination and Excessive Thirst:

Elevated blood sugar levels can lead to increased urine production, causing frequent urination. Consequently, excessive fluid loss can result in heightened thirst as the body attempts to maintain hydration. These symptoms are often early warning signs that prompt individuals to consult healthcare professionals for further evaluation.

Blurred Vision:

Changes in vision, such as blurred vision, can occur when high blood sugar levels affect the lens of the eye. While this symptom is not exclusive to diabetes, it can serve as an indicator, especially when accompanied by other diabetes-related symptoms.

Slow Wound Healing:

Type-2 diabetes can impact the body's ability to heal wounds and injuries. Impaired circulation and compromised immune function contribute to delayed wound healing, making individuals with diabetes more susceptible to infections.

Diagnostic Tests:

Diagnosing type-2 diabetes involves various tests aimed at assessing blood sugar levels and overall metabolic health. Fasting blood sugar tests, oral glucose tolerance tests (OGTT), and hemoglobin A1c tests are commonly employed to diagnose and monitor diabetes.

- **Fasting Blood Sugar Test:** This test measures blood sugar levels after an overnight fast. Elevated fasting blood sugar levels may indicate diabetes.

- **Oral Glucose Tolerance Test (OGTT):** This involves fasting overnight and then drinking a glucose solution. Blood sugar levels are measured at intervals to assess how the body processes glucose. Elevated readings may indicate diabetes.

- **Hemoglobin A1c Test:** This test provides an average of blood sugar levels over the past two to three months. It offers a comprehensive view of long-term glucose control.

Importance of Early Diagnosis:

Early diagnosis of type-2 diabetes is crucial for preventing complications and initiating timely interventions. Uncontrolled diabetes can lead to serious health issues, including cardiovascular disease, kidney damage, nerve damage, and vision problems. Detecting diabetes in its early stages allows individuals to implement lifestyle changes, medication, and other interventions to manage the condition effectively.

2.3 Complications Associated with Type-2 Diabetes

Type-2 diabetes, when left unmanaged, can lead to a range of complications affecting various organ systems. Understanding these potential complications underscores the importance of proactive diabetes management to preserve overall health and well-being.

Cardiovascular Complications:

Cardiovascular disease is a major concern for individuals with type-2 diabetes. Elevated blood sugar levels contribute to the accumulation of plaque in blood vessels, increasing the risk of heart attacks and strokes. Additionally, diabetes can lead to high blood pressure and abnormal cholesterol levels, further amplifying cardiovascular risks. Lifestyle modifications, including a heart-healthy diet and regular exercise, play a crucial role in mitigating these risks.

Kidney Damage (Nephropathy):

The kidneys are vulnerable to damage in individuals with diabetes. Persistent high blood sugar levels can lead to nephropathy, a condition characterized by impaired kidney function. Early stages may manifest as protein in the urine (proteinuria), while advanced stages can progress to chronic kidney disease (CKD). Regular monitoring of kidney function through blood and urine tests is essential for timely intervention.

Neuropathy (Nerve Damage):

Nerve damage, or neuropathy, is a common complication of diabetes. It can manifest as tingling, numbness, or pain, usually starting in the extremities. Neuropathy can affect both sensory and motor nerves, leading to complications such as foot ulcers and difficulty in coordinating movements. Comprehensive foot care, blood sugar control, and medication management are crucial in preventing and managing diabetic neuropathy.

Retinopathy (Eye Complications):

Diabetes can impact the eyes, leading to a condition known as diabetic retinopathy. Elevated blood sugar levels cause damage to the blood vessels in the retina, potentially leading to vision impairment and blindness if left untreated. Regular eye examinations and blood sugar control are essential in preventing and managing diabetic retinopathy.

Foot Complications:

Diabetes can affect circulation and sensation in the feet, making individuals more susceptible to foot problems. Poor circulation can lead to slow wound healing, while nerve damage may result in reduced sensation, making it challenging to detect injuries. Proper foot care, regular examinations, and appropriate footwear are crucial in preventing complications such as infections and ulcers.

Infections and Slow Healing:

Individuals with diabetes are more prone to infections due to compromised immune function. High blood sugar levels create an environment conducive to bacterial and fungal growth. Wound healing is also impaired in diabetes, increasing the risk of infections. Vigilant hygiene practices, prompt wound care, and blood sugar control are essential in preventing and managing infections.

Mental Health Implications:

Living with a chronic condition like type-2 diabetes can take a toll on mental health. The constant management efforts, concerns about complications, and lifestyle adjustments may contribute to stress, anxiety, and depression. Recognizing the mental health implications

17

of diabetes and seeking appropriate support, including counseling and support groups, is integral to comprehensive diabetes care.

Preventive Measures and Management Strategies:

While the potential complications associated with type-2 diabetes are significant, adopting preventive measures and effective management strategies can mitigate these risks. Comprehensive diabetes care involves regular monitoring of blood sugar levels, adherence to prescribed medications, a balanced diet, regular physical activity, and routine medical check-ups.

CHAPTER 3

NUTRITIONAL GUIDELINES FOR TYPE-2 DIABETES

3.1 Importance of Balanced Nutrition

Balanced nutrition is the cornerstone of effective management for individuals with type-2 diabetes. The significance of maintaining a well-rounded diet cannot be overstated, as it directly influences blood sugar control, weight management, and overall health. Achieving balance involves thoughtful consideration of macronutrients, portion control, and mindful food choices.

Role of Balanced Nutrition:

Balanced nutrition is vital for individuals with type-2 diabetes as it aims to achieve several key objectives. Primarily, it helps in regulating blood sugar levels by providing a steady supply of carbohydrates that are absorbed gradually. This prevents sharp spikes in blood sugar, promoting stable energy levels throughout the day.

Furthermore, a balanced diet supports weight management, a crucial aspect of diabetes care. Maintaining a healthy weight contributes to improved insulin sensitivity, reducing the strain on the pancreas to produce excess insulin. This, in turn, helps in better blood sugar control and lowers the risk of complications associated with obesity.

Balanced nutrition also ensures an adequate intake of essential nutrients, including vitamins, minerals, and fiber. These nutrients play a crucial role in overall well-being and can contribute to the prevention of complications associated with diabetes, such as cardiovascular disease and nerve damage.

Components of a Balanced Diet:

A balanced diet for individuals with type-2 diabetes should include a variety of nutrient-dense foods. The key components include:

- **Carbohydrates:** Choosing complex carbohydrates with a low glycemic index is essential. Whole grains, legumes, and fibrous vegetables provide sustained energy without causing rapid spikes in blood sugar. Portion control is equally crucial, ensuring a moderate intake of carbohydrates at each meal.
- **Proteins:** Including lean protein sources such as poultry, fish, tofu, legumes, and low-fat dairy supports muscle maintenance and satiety. Protein

20

intake should be distributed evenly throughout the day to aid in blood sugar control.

- **Fats:** Opting for healthy fats, such as those found in avocados, nuts, seeds, and olive oil, is essential. Limiting saturated and trans fats helps in managing cholesterol levels and reducing the risk of cardiovascular complications.

- **Fruits and Vegetables:** These should form a substantial portion of the diet. Rich in vitamins, minerals, and fiber, fruits and vegetables contribute to overall health. While they contain carbohydrates, the fiber content helps in gradual glucose absorption.

- **Portion Control:** Controlling portion sizes is critical in preventing overconsumption of calories and carbohydrates. Measuring food portions, using smaller plates, and being mindful of portion sizes during meals contribute to better blood sugar management.

Meal Timing and Frequency:

In addition to considering food choices, meal timing and frequency play a crucial role in achieving balanced nutrition. Spreading meals throughout the day, with regular intervals, helps in preventing sharp fluctuations in blood sugar levels. Including snacks that combine protein and fiber can be particularly beneficial in maintaining stable energy levels between meals.

Importance of Individualization:

While general guidelines provide a foundation for balanced nutrition, it's crucial to recognize the importance of individualization. Each person's response to different foods varies, and factors such as age, activity level, and medication use influence dietary requirements. Regular monitoring of blood sugar levels and consultation with healthcare professionals can help tailor nutritional recommendations to meet individual needs.

3.2 Recommended Daily Allowances

Understanding the recommended daily allowances (RDAs) for various nutrients is pivotal for individuals with type-2 diabetes. Meeting these allowances through a well-planned and balanced diet ensures the body receives the necessary nutrients for optimal functioning, supporting overall health and diabetes management.

Caloric Intake and Energy Needs:

The total caloric intake for individuals with type-2 diabetes depends on various factors, including age, gender, weight, activity level, and overall health goals. While there is no one-size-fits-all approach, it's essential to strike a balance that supports weight management and blood sugar control.

Determining individual energy needs involves considering factors such as basal metabolic rate (BMR) and physical activity level. BMR represents the calories required for basic bodily functions at rest, while physical activity contributes to additional energy expenditure. Achieving a balance between caloric intake and expenditure is crucial for weight maintenance and blood sugar control.

Carbohydrates:

Carbohydrates have a direct impact on blood sugar levels, making their intake a focal point in diabetes management. The recommended daily allowance for carbohydrates varies, but a general guideline is to aim for 45-65% of total daily calories. Choosing complex carbohydrates with a low glycemic index and distributing them evenly throughout meals supports stable blood sugar levels.

Proteins:

Protein requirements depend on factors such as age, activity level, and overall health. The recommended daily allowance for protein is approximately 0.8 grams per kilogram of body weight for adults. Including lean protein sources in each meal and snack helps in muscle maintenance, satiety, and blood sugar control.

Fats:

The recommended daily allowance for fats is typically around 20-35% of total daily calories. It's essential to focus on healthy fats, including monounsaturated and polyunsaturated fats, while limiting saturated and trans fats. Including sources such as avocados, nuts, seeds, and olive oil contributes to heart health and overall well-being.

Vitamins and Minerals:

Meeting the recommended daily allowances for vitamins and minerals is crucial for overall health. Nutrient-dense foods, including fruits, vegetables, whole grains, and lean proteins, provide essential vitamins and minerals. In some cases, supplementation may be recommended, especially for nutrients like vitamin D, vitamin B12, and iron.

Fiber:

Fiber plays a vital role in digestive health and blood sugar control. The recommended daily allowance for fiber is around 25 grams for women and 38 grams for men. Including a variety of fruits, vegetables, whole grains, and legumes helps in achieving adequate fiber intake.

Hydration:

Adequate hydration is often overlooked but is integral to overall health. The recommended daily allowance for fluid intake varies, but a general guideline is to aim for about 8 cups (64 ounces) of water per day. Staying well-hydrated supports kidney function, digestion, and overall well-being.

Individualization and Monitoring:

While RDAs provide general guidelines, individualization is key in diabetes management. Factors such as age, gender, activity level, and medication use influence nutritional needs. Regular monitoring of blood sugar levels and consultation with healthcare professionals help tailor dietary recommendations to meet individual requirements.

3.3 Monitoring Blood Sugar Levels

Monitoring blood sugar levels is a fundamental aspect of diabetes management, empowering individuals to make informed decisions about their diet, medication, and overall lifestyle. Regular monitoring provides valuable insights into how the body responds to different foods, activities, and medications, enabling proactive measures to maintain optimal blood sugar control.

Importance of Blood Sugar Monitoring:

Monitoring blood sugar levels is essential for several reasons:

- **Dietary Management:** Understanding the impact of different foods on blood sugar levels helps individuals make informed dietary choices. Monitoring allows for the identification of foods that cause spikes and the adjustment of portion sizes to maintain stable blood sugar levels.

- **Medication Adjustment:** For individuals on oral medications or insulin, regular monitoring guides medication adjustments. This is particularly crucial as medication needs may vary based on factors such as activity level, stress, illness, and changes in diet.

- **Identification of Patterns:** Regular monitoring reveals patterns in blood sugar fluctuations, aiding in the identification of trends. This includes recognizing how the body responds to meals, the influence of physical activity, and the impact of stress on blood sugar levels.

- **Prevention of Complications:** Consistent blood sugar monitoring contributes to the prevention of complications associated with diabetes. Maintaining optimal blood sugar control reduces the risk of cardiovascular disease, kidney damage, nerve damage, and other diabetes-related complications.

- *Methods of Blood Sugar Monitoring:* There are various methods for monitoring blood sugar levels, each offering unique advantages:

- **Self-Monitoring of Blood Glucose (SMBG):** This involves using a glucometer to measure blood sugar levels at home. Regular testing, typically before meals and at specific intervals throughout the day, provides real-time information on blood sugar control.

- **Continuous Glucose Monitoring (CGM):** CGM systems involve the use of a small sensor placed under the skin to continuously monitor glucose levels. This technology provides a comprehensive view of blood sugar trends over time, offering valuable insights into daily patterns.

- **Hemoglobin A1c Testing:** This blood test provides an average of blood sugar levels over the past two to three months. While not a substitute for daily monitoring, it offers a broader perspective on long-term glucose control.

Frequency of Monitoring:

The frequency of blood sugar monitoring varies among individuals and may be influenced by factors such as the type of diabetes, treatment plan, and overall health. For some, monitoring may be recommended multiple times a day, especially if on insulin therapy. Others may benefit from less frequent monitoring based on their diabetes management plan.

Interpreting Blood Sugar Readings:

Interpreting blood sugar readings involves understanding target ranges and the significance of various values:

Fasting Blood Sugar: Ideally, fasting blood sugar levels before meals should fall within the range of 80-130 mg/dL. This provides a baseline measurement before the intake of food.

Postprandial Blood Sugar: Postprandial (after-meal) blood sugar levels are typically recommended to be below 180 mg/dL two hours after eating. This helps assess the impact of meals on blood sugar.

Hemoglobin A1c Levels: The target Hemoglobin A1c level is often set below 7%. This reflects an average blood sugar level over the past two to three months.

Utilizing Monitoring Data:

The data obtained through blood sugar monitoring serves as a valuable tool in diabetes self-management:

Dietary Adjustments: Identifying how different foods affect blood sugar levels allows for dietary adjustments. This includes modifying portion sizes, choosing lower-glycemic options, and spreading carbohydrate intake evenly throughout the day.

Medication Management: For individuals on medication, monitoring helps in adjusting medication doses based on daily variations in blood sugar levels. This is particularly important to prevent hypoglycemia (low blood sugar) or hyperglycemia (high blood sugar).

Lifestyle Modifications: Recognizing patterns in blood sugar fluctuations informs lifestyle modifications. This includes adjusting physical activity levels, managing stress, and addressing factors that contribute to blood sugar variability.

Communication with Healthcare Professionals: Sharing monitoring data with healthcare professionals during regular check-ups facilitates collaborative decision-making. Adjustments to the diabetes management plan can be made based on the insights gained from monitoring.

Challenges and Coping Strategies:

While blood sugar monitoring is essential, it can pose challenges, including the fear of needles, inconvenience, or emotional stress associated with fluctuations in readings. Coping strategies include:

- **Education and Support:** Comprehensive education on the importance of monitoring and its role in diabetes management helps individuals overcome fears. Support groups and counseling can provide emotional support.

- **Integration into Daily Routine:** Incorporating monitoring into daily routines makes it a more manageable task. Setting reminders, using smartphone apps, and establishing a consistent schedule contribute to adherence.

- **Mindful Interpretation:** It's crucial to approach blood sugar readings with a mindset of learning rather than judgment. Each reading provides an opportunity to understand the body's response and make informed adjustments.

CHAPTER 4

BUILDING A HEALTHY PLATE

4.1 Portion Control

Portion control is a fundamental aspect of managing type-2 diabetes and promoting overall health. It involves being mindful of the quantity of food consumed at each meal and snack, a practice that contributes to better blood sugar control, weight management, and overall well-being.

Understanding Portion Sizes:

In a world where oversized portions have become the norm, understanding appropriate portion sizes is essential. Portion control is not about deprivation but rather about consuming the right amount of nutrients to meet the body's needs without excessive caloric intake. It's about quality over quantity.

One effective way to visualize appropriate portions is by using everyday objects as a reference. For example, a serving of meat should be about the size of a deck of cards, a cup of vegetables is approximately the size of a baseball, and a tablespoon of oil is comparable to the tip of your thumb. These visual cues help individuals gauge portions without relying on measuring tools.

Benefits of Portion Control:

1. **Blood Sugar Control:** Controlling portion sizes helps manage blood sugar levels more effectively. Smaller, well-balanced meals prevent sharp spikes in blood sugar, promoting stable glucose levels throughout the day.

2. **Weight Management:** Portion control plays a pivotal role in weight management. Overeating, even on healthy foods, can contribute to excess calorie intake. By moderating portion sizes, individuals can achieve and maintain a healthy weight, reducing the risk of obesity-related complications.

3. **Digestive Health:** Proper portion control supports digestive health. Overeating can strain the digestive system, leading to issues such as indigestion and discomfort. Smaller, well-distributed meals facilitate better digestion.

4. **Energy Levels:** Consuming appropriately sized portions ensures a steady supply of energy without causing energy crashes or lethargy. This is particularly important for individuals with type-2

diabetes, as stable energy levels contribute to better blood sugar management.

Practical Tips for Portion Control:

1. **Use Smaller Plates:** Opting for smaller plates creates the illusion of a fuller plate, promoting satisfaction with smaller portions.

2. **Be Mindful of Snacking:** Snacking can contribute significantly to overall caloric intake. Instead of mindless snacking, portion out snacks in advance and avoid eating directly from large packages.

3. **Read Nutrition Labels:** Understanding serving sizes on nutrition labels helps in making informed choices. Pay attention to portion sizes listed and adjust accordingly.

4. **Listen to Hunger and Fullness Cues:** Being in tune with the body's hunger and fullness cues is crucial. Eating slowly and savoring each bite allows for better recognition of satiety.

5. **Divide Restaurant Portions:** Restaurant servings are often larger than necessary. Consider splitting a dish with a dining companion or requesting a to-go box to portion out a portion before starting the meal.

6. **Stay Hydrated:** Drinking water before meals helps create a sense of fullness, preventing overeating. Additionally, thirst can sometimes be mistaken for hunger.

7. **Practice the Plate Method:** Divide the plate into sections for different food groups – half the plate for non-starchy vegetables, one-quarter for lean protein, and one-quarter for whole grains or starchy vegetables.

Portion control is a simple yet powerful tool for managing type-2 diabetes and promoting overall health. By adopting mindful eating habits and being aware of portion sizes, individuals can take control of their nutrition and optimize their well-being.

4.2 Balancing Carbohydrates, Proteins, and Fats

Achieving a harmonious balance between carbohydrates, proteins, and fats is essential for individuals with type-2 diabetes. This balance not only contributes to better blood sugar control but also supports overall health and well-being. Understanding the role of each macronutrient and making thoughtful choices fosters a well-rounded and diabetes-friendly diet.

Balancing Carbohydrates:

Carbohydrates have a direct impact on blood sugar levels, making their management a key focus for individuals with type-2 diabetes. However, it's important to recognize that not all carbohydrates are created equal. The focus should be on choosing complex carbohydrates with a low glycemic index (GI) that provide sustained energy without causing rapid spikes in blood sugar.

- **Whole Grains:** Opt for whole grains such as brown rice, quinoa, whole wheat, and oats. These grains contain fiber, which slows down the absorption of glucose, promoting stable blood sugar levels.
- **Legumes:** Beans, lentils, and peas are excellent sources of complex carbohydrates and fiber. Including these in meals contributes to satiety and supports blood sugar control.
- **Fruits:** While fruits contain natural sugars, they also provide essential vitamins, minerals, and fiber. Choosing whole fruits over fruit juices and incorporating a variety of fruits into the diet is beneficial.

Balancing Proteins:

Proteins play a crucial role in maintaining muscle mass, supporting satiety, and aiding in blood sugar control. It's essential to include lean protein sources while considering individual dietary preferences and health goals.

- **Poultry and Lean Meats:** Skinless poultry, lean cuts of meat, and fish are excellent sources of protein. Grilling, baking, or broiling these protein sources helps in minimizing added fats.

- **Plant-Based Proteins:** Tofu, tempeh, legumes, and plant-based protein sources offer alternatives for individuals following vegetarian or vegan diets. These options provide essential amino acids and contribute to a well-balanced plate.

- **Dairy or Dairy Alternatives:** Low-fat or fat-free dairy products, as well as fortified dairy alternatives, contribute to protein intake while also providing essential nutrients like calcium and vitamin D.

Balancing Fats:

While fats have often been stigmatized, it's crucial to differentiate between healthy fats and those that contribute to health issues. Including sources of healthy fats in the diet is essential for cardiovascular health and overall well-being.

- **Monounsaturated Fats:** Olive oil, avocados, and nuts are rich in monounsaturated fats. These fats contribute to heart health and can be included in moderation as part of a diabetes-friendly diet.

- **Polyunsaturated Fats:** Fatty fish, flaxseeds, chia seeds, and walnuts are sources of polyunsaturated fats, including omega-3 fatty acids. These fats have anti-inflammatory properties and support cardiovascular health.

- **Limiting Saturated and Trans Fats:** Saturated and trans fats, often found in processed and fried foods, should be limited. These fats can contribute to insulin resistance and increase the risk of cardiovascular complications.

Practical Tips for Balancing Macronutrients:

- **Create Balanced Meals:** Aim to create meals that include a balance of carbohydrates, proteins, and fats. The plate method, dividing the plate into sections for each macronutrient, can serve as a practical guide.

- **Consider Glycemic Index:** Understanding the glycemic index of foods helps in choosing carbohydrates that have a minimal impact on blood sugar levels. Combining low-GI carbohydrates with proteins and fats supports balanced meals.
- **Snack Wisely:** When snacking, consider combining a carbohydrate with a protein or healthy fat. For example, pairing apple slices with almond butter provides a satisfying and balanced snack.
- **Choose Whole, Unprocessed Foods:** Whole, unprocessed foods naturally contain a balance of macronutrients. Choosing foods in their whole form, such as fruits, vegetables, and lean proteins, supports a balanced diet.
- **Mindful Eating:** Practicing mindful eating involves paying attention to hunger and fullness cues. This approach helps in making conscious choices about portion sizes and macronutrient distribution.

4.3 Choosing the Right Foods

The journey to building a healthy plate for individuals with type-2 diabetes involves making thoughtful choices about the types of foods consumed. By focusing on nutrient-dense options, emphasizing variety, and considering individual dietary preferences, individuals can create a well-rounded and diabetes-friendly eating plan.

Prioritizing Nutrient-Dense Foods:

Nutrient density refers to the concentration of essential nutrients per calorie in a given food. Choosing nutrient-dense foods ensures that the body receives a rich supply of vitamins, minerals, and other vital components without excessive caloric intake.

- **Non-Starchy Vegetables:** Non-starchy vegetables such as leafy greens, broccoli, cauliflower, and peppers are low in calories and high in nutrients. They provide fiber, vitamins, and minerals without significantly impacting blood sugar levels.

- **Whole Fruits:** While fruits contain natural sugars, they also offer a plethora of nutrients and fiber. Choosing whole fruits over fruit juices and processed snacks supports overall health.

- **Lean Proteins:** Including lean protein sources such as poultry, fish, tofu, legumes, and low-fat dairy promotes muscle maintenance, satiety, and stable blood sugar levels.

- **Whole Grains:** Whole grains such as quinoa, brown rice, oats, and whole wheat provide complex carbohydrates, fiber, and essential nutrients. These grains contribute to sustained energy levels and support digestive health.
- **Healthy Fats:** Opting for sources of healthy fats, including avocados, nuts, seeds, and olive oil, contributes to cardiovascular health and overall well-being.
- **Dairy or Dairy Alternatives:** Low-fat or fat-free dairy products, as well as fortified dairy alternatives, offer a source of calcium, vitamin D, and protein.
- **Herbs and Spices:** Herbs and spices not only add flavor to meals without extra calories but also offer potential health benefits. Some spices, such as cinnamon, have been associated with improved insulin sensitivity.

Emphasizing Variety:

Variety in food choices ensures a broad spectrum of nutrients and enhances the overall eating experience. Including a diverse range of foods from different food groups promotes optimal nutrition and prevents monotony in the diet.

- **Colorful Vegetables and Fruits:** The vibrant colors of fruits and vegetables are often indicative of different nutrients. Including a variety of colors in the diet ensures a diverse array of vitamins, minerals, and antioxidants.

- **Protein Variety:** Incorporating a variety of protein sources, including plant-based options, supports diverse amino acid profiles. This not only contributes to better nutrition but also caters to individual dietary preferences.

- **Whole Grain Options:** Choosing different whole grains provides a range of nutrients and flavors. Experimenting with grains such as quinoa, barley, and farro introduces variety and nutritional benefits.

- **Exploring Different Cooking Methods:** Varying cooking methods, such as steaming, roasting, grilling, and sautéing, adds diversity to meals. Each method imparts unique textures and flavors to ingredients.

- **Incorporating Herbs and Spices:** Experimenting with different herbs and spices enhances the taste of dishes without relying on excessive salt, sugar, or unhealthy fats. Additionally, some spices may offer health benefits.

Considering Individual Dietary Preferences:

Adopting a diabetes-friendly eating plan doesn't mean sacrificing personal preferences or cultural influences. It's essential to tailor dietary choices to individual tastes while making informed decisions about portion sizes and nutrient balance.

- **Flexibility with Carbohydrates:** Recognizing that different individuals may tolerate carbohydrates differently, it's essential to personalize carbohydrate intake. Some may benefit from a lower-carbohydrate approach, while others can include a moderate amount in their diets.

- **Plant-Based Options:** For those following vegetarian or vegan diets, incorporating a variety of plant-based proteins, legumes, and whole grains ensures adequate nutrition. Plant-based diets can be diabetes-friendly with careful attention to nutrient balance.

- **Cultural Considerations:** Embracing cultural food preferences is integral to long-term adherence to a diabetes-friendly diet. By modifying traditional recipes to include healthier ingredients or adjusting portion sizes, individuals can enjoy the flavors of their cultural cuisines.

- **Personalizing Protein Sources:** While lean animal proteins are a common choice, individuals can explore alternative protein sources based on personal preferences. Plant-based proteins, dairy, and fish provide diverse options.

Practical Tips for Choosing the Right Foods:

- **Meal Planning:** Planning meals in advance allows for thoughtful consideration of nutrient balance. This includes incorporating a variety of foods from different food groups.
- **Grocery Shopping with a List:** Having a shopping list helps in focusing on nutrient-dense foods and avoiding impulsive purchases of less healthy options.
- **Label Reading:** Understanding food labels aids in making informed choices. Paying attention to serving sizes, nutrient content, and ingredient lists contributes to better decision-making.
- **Mindful Eating Practices:** Practicing mindful eating involves savoring each bite, paying attention to hunger and fullness cues, and

appreciating the sensory aspects of food. This approach supports healthy food choices.

- **Experimenting with New Foods:** Trying new foods and recipes introduces variety into the diet. It can also be an enjoyable way to discover new flavors and textures.

Building a healthy plate for individuals with type-2 diabetes involves choosing nutrient-dense foods, emphasizing variety, and considering individual preferences. By making thoughtful and informed choices, individuals can create a sustainable and diabetes-friendly eating plan that promotes optimal health and well-being.

CHAPTER 5

TYPE-2 DIABETES FOOD LIST

5.1 Foods to Include

A well-planned and balanced diet is crucial for managing Type-2 diabetes. Including the right foods can contribute to stable blood sugar levels, weight management, and overall well-being. This section explores the key categories of foods to include in the diet for individuals with Type-2 diabetes.

Whole Grains and Fiber-rich Foods

Whole grains and fiber-rich foods play a pivotal role in the diet for Type-2 diabetes. They provide sustained energy, contribute to stable blood sugar levels, and offer a range of essential nutrients.

Examples of Whole Grains:

- **Quinoa:** Quinoa is a versatile whole grain that is rich in protein, fiber, and various vitamins and minerals. It has a lower glycemic index compared to some other grains, making it a favorable choice for individuals with diabetes.

- **Brown Rice:** Brown rice is a whole grain that retains its bran and germ layers, providing more fiber, vitamins, and minerals compared to white rice. It is a complex carbohydrate that is absorbed more slowly, helping in blood sugar control.

- **Oats:** Oats are high in soluble fiber, known to help regulate blood sugar levels. They also contain beta-glucans, which contribute to heart health. Choose whole oats or steel-cut oats for maximum nutritional benefits.

- **Whole Wheat:** Whether in the form of whole wheat bread, pasta, or flour, choosing whole wheat options ensures a higher fiber content and a slower release of glucose into the bloodstream.

- **Barley:** Barley is rich in both soluble and insoluble fiber, providing a range of health benefits. It can be used in soups, stews, or as a side dish.

Benefits of Whole Grains and Fiber:

- **Blood Sugar Control:** The fiber in whole grains slows down the digestion and absorption of carbohydrates, preventing rapid spikes in blood sugar levels.

- **Weight Management:** High-fiber foods contribute to a feeling of fullness, promoting weight management by reducing overeating.

- **Heart Health:** The soluble fiber in oats, barley, and other whole grains helps lower cholesterol levels, reducing the risk of cardiovascular complications associated with Type-2 diabetes.
- **Digestive Health:** Insoluble fiber supports digestive health by preventing constipation and promoting regular bowel movements.

Practical Tips:

- **Choose Whole Grains:** Opt for whole grains such as brown rice, quinoa, and whole wheat bread over refined grains.
- **Read Labels:** When selecting packaged foods, read labels to ensure they contain whole grains and are not overly processed.
- **Experiment with Different Grains:** Explore a variety of whole grains to add diversity to your diet. Try incorporating ancient grains like farro, freekeh, or millet.
- **Combine with Lean Proteins:** Create balanced meals by combining whole grains with lean proteins and plenty of non-starchy vegetables.

Lean Proteins

- Lean proteins are essential components of a diabetes-friendly diet. They provide necessary amino acids for muscle maintenance, contribute to satiety, and have minimal impact on blood sugar levels.

Examples of Lean Proteins:

- **Poultry:** Skinless chicken or turkey breasts are excellent sources of lean protein. They can be grilled, baked, or sautéed for a healthy and delicious meal.

- **Fish:** Fatty fish like salmon, mackerel, and trout are rich in omega-3 fatty acids. These healthy fats offer cardiovascular benefits and support overall health.

- **Tofu and Tempeh:** Plant-based protein sources like tofu and tempeh provide alternatives for those following vegetarian or vegan diets. They are versatile and can be used in various dishes.

- **Legumes:** Beans, lentils, and chickpeas are high in protein and fiber. They also have a low glycemic index, making them excellent choices for blood sugar control.

- **Lean Cuts of Meat:** Opt for lean cuts of beef or pork, such as sirloin or tenderloin. Trim visible fats before cooking to reduce saturated fat intake.

Benefits of Lean Proteins:

- **Blood Sugar Control:** Lean proteins have minimal impact on blood sugar levels, making them suitable choices for individuals with Type-2 diabetes.
- **Muscle Maintenance:** Protein is essential for maintaining muscle mass, especially important for overall health and metabolism.
- **Satiety:** Including lean proteins in meals promotes a feeling of fullness, reducing the likelihood of overeating.
- **Nutrient Density:** Lean proteins provide essential nutrients like iron, zinc, and B vitamins without excessive saturated fat.

Practical Tips:

- **Diversify Protein Sources:** Include a variety of protein sources in your diet to ensure a broad spectrum of nutrients. Mix up your choices with both animal and plant-based options.

- **Practice Healthy Cooking Methods:** Opt for grilling, baking, broiling, or steaming when preparing proteins to minimize added fats.
- **Portion Control:** Be mindful of portion sizes, as excessive protein intake can contribute to calorie consumption. Aim for a palm-sized portion of protein at each meal.
- **Combine with Vegetables:** Create balanced meals by combining lean proteins with a generous serving of non-starchy vegetables.

Fruits and Vegetables

Fruits and vegetables are foundational elements of a diabetes-friendly diet. They are rich in fiber, vitamins, minerals, and antioxidants while being low in calories.

Examples of Fruits:

- **Berries:** Blueberries, strawberries, raspberries, and blackberries are not only delicious but also packed with antioxidants and fiber.
- **Apples:** Apples are a good source of soluble fiber, particularly in the form of pectin, which aids in blood sugar regulation.

- **Citrus Fruits:** Oranges, grapefruits, lemons, and limes provide vitamin C and fiber. They also have a low glycemic index.
- **Pears:** Pears offer dietary fiber, including both soluble and insoluble types, contributing to digestive health.
- **Cherries:** Cherries contain anthocyanins, which may have anti-inflammatory and antioxidant effects.

Examples of Vegetables:

Leafy Greens: Spinach, kale, Swiss chard, and collard greens are rich in vitamins, minerals, and antioxidants.

Cruciferous Vegetables: Broccoli, cauliflower, Brussels sprouts, and cabbage are high in fiber and offer potential anti-cancer benefits.

Colorful Vegetables: Bell peppers, carrots, tomatoes, and sweet potatoes provide a range of nutrients and add vibrant colors to meals.

Zucchini and Eggplant: These vegetables are low in calories and can be versatile additions to various dishes.

Asparagus: Asparagus is a good source of fiber, folate, and vitamins A and C.

Benefits of Fruits and Vegetables:

- **Fiber Content:** The fiber in fruits and vegetables contributes to satiety, digestive health, and blood sugar control.
- **Nutrient Density:** Fruits and vegetables are rich in essential vitamins, minerals, and antioxidants with minimal impact on blood sugar levels.
- **Weight Management:** The low-calorie density of fruits and vegetables makes them valuable for weight management.
- **Heart Health:** The potassium, fiber, and antioxidants in these foods contribute to cardiovascular health.

Practical Tips:

- **Embrace Variety:** Include a colorful variety of fruits and vegetables to ensure a broad spectrum of nutrients.
- **Mindful Eating:** Practice mindful eating by savoring the flavors and textures of fruits and vegetables. This promotes a positive relationship with food.
- **Explore Different Cooking Methods:** Experiment with various cooking methods such as

roasting, steaming, sautéing, and grilling to enhance the taste and texture of fruits and vegetables.

- **Incorporate as Snacks:** Fruits and vegetables make excellent snacks. Keep pre-cut options in the refrigerator for convenient and healthy choices.

Healthy Fats

Healthy fats are an integral part of a diabetes-friendly diet. They provide essential fatty acids, support heart health, and contribute to overall well-being.

Examples of Healthy Fats:

- **Avocado:** Avocado is rich in monounsaturated fats, which have been associated with improved insulin sensitivity.
- **Nuts:** Almonds, walnuts, and pistachios provide healthy fats, fiber, and various vitamins and minerals.
- **Seeds:** Flaxseeds, chia seeds, and sunflower seeds are sources of omega-3 fatty acids, fiber, and essential nutrients.

- **Olive Oil:** Extra virgin olive oil is a staple in the Mediterranean diet, known for its heart-protective benefits.
- **Fatty Fish:** Salmon, mackerel, trout, and sardines are rich in omega-3 fatty acids, promoting cardiovascular health.

Benefits of Healthy Fats:

- **Heart Health:** Monounsaturated and polyunsaturated fats contribute to heart health by reducing cholesterol levels and inflammation.
- **Insulin Sensitivity:** Certain healthy fats, such as those found in avocados and olive oil, may improve insulin sensitivity.
- **Satiety:** Including healthy fats in meals promotes a feeling of fullness, reducing the likelihood of overeating.
- **Brain Health:** Omega-3 fatty acids, found in fatty fish and certain seeds, are essential for brain health and cognitive function.

Practical Tips:

- **Moderation is Key:** While healthy fats offer benefits, moderation is crucial. Be mindful of portion sizes to avoid excess calorie intake.

- **Diversify Fat Sources:** Include a variety of sources of healthy fats in your diet for a well-rounded nutrient profile.

- **Use Olive Oil in Cooking:** Substitute butter or other cooking oils with extra virgin olive oil when preparing meals.

- **Snack on Nuts and Seeds:** Choose nuts and seeds as satisfying snacks, but be mindful of portion sizes due to their calorie density.

5.2 Foods to Limit

While certain foods are beneficial for individuals with Type-2 diabetes, others should be consumed in moderation or limited to maintain optimal blood sugar control and overall health. This section explores categories of foods that individuals with Type-2 diabetes should be mindful of.

High-Glycomic Indox Foods

High-Glycemic Index (GI) foods are those that cause a rapid spike in blood sugar levels when consumed. Managing the intake of these foods is crucial for individuals with Type-2 diabetes to prevent abrupt increases in glucose levels.

Examples of High-Glycemic Index Foods:

- **White Bread:** Refined grains, such as white bread, have a high GI, causing a quick rise in blood sugar levels.
- **White Rice:** White rice, stripped of its bran and germ layers, has a higher GI compared to brown rice.
- **Potatoes:** Potatoes, especially when mashed or processed, have a high GI due to their quick conversion to glucose.
- **Sugary Cereals:** Breakfast cereals with added sugars and low fiber content can have a high impact on blood sugar.
- **Instant Oatmeal:** Some instant oatmeal varieties may have added sugars and lack the fiber present in whole oats.

Managing High-Glycemic Index Foods:

- **Combine with Fiber:** Pairing high-GI foods with fiber-rich options can help slow down the absorption of glucose.
- **Monitor Portion Sizes:** Be mindful of portion sizes, especially when consuming high-GI foods, to avoid excessive spikes in blood sugar levels.

- **Choose Whole Grains:** Opt for whole grains with a lower GI, such as brown rice or quinoa, instead of refined grains.

Processed and Sugary Foods

Processed and sugary foods contribute to excess calorie intake, may lead to weight gain, and can negatively impact blood sugar control. Limiting the consumption of these foods is crucial for managing Type-2 diabetes.

Examples of Processed and Sugary Foods:

- **Sodas and Sugary Drinks:** Beverages with added sugars, including sodas, energy drinks, and sweetened teas, can lead to rapid increases in blood sugar.
- **Candies and Sweets:** Confections with high sugar content, such as candies, cookies, and pastries, should be consumed sparingly.
- **Sweetened Breakfast Cereals:** Cereals with added sugars contribute to elevated blood sugar levels and are often low in nutritional value.
- **Processed Snacks:** Chips, crackers, and other processed snacks may contain unhealthy fats and high levels of sodium, impacting overall health.

- **Sweetened Yogurts:** Some flavored yogurts have added sugars, which can affect blood sugar levels. Choose plain yogurt and add your own fruit for sweetness.

Sodium and Type-2 Diabetes

While sodium itself doesn't directly impact blood sugar levels, excessive sodium intake can contribute to other health issues that individuals with type-2 diabetes may be more susceptible to, such as high blood pressure and cardiovascular disease.

Canned and Processed Foods: Canned soups, processed meats, and certain convenience foods can be high in sodium. Choose fresh or homemade alternatives when possible.

Restaurant and Fast Food: Restaurant and fast-food meals often contain high levels of sodium. Opt for healthier, homemade meals with less added salt.

Condiments and Sauces: Some condiments and sauces, including ketchup, soy sauce, and salad dressings, can be sources of hidden sodium. Choose low-sodium versions or make homemade alternatives.

Frozen Dinners: Pre-packaged frozen dinners can be convenient but are often high in sodium. Consider preparing and freezing homemade meals with lower salt content.

In conclusion, a well-considered food list is a valuable tool for individuals managing type-2 diabetes. By focusing on nutrient-dense foods, incorporating a variety of whole grains, lean proteins, fruits, and vegetables, and limiting processed and sugary items, individuals can create a balanced and health-promoting diet that supports diabetes management and overall well-being.

NON-STARCHY VEGETABLES

Below is a table featuring 50 non-starchy vegetables suitable for individuals with type-2 diabetes. The table includes information on food type, portion sizes, approximate glycemic index (GI) values (measured on a scale of 0 to 100), and basic nutritional information per 100 grams.

Food Type	Portion Size	Low Glycemic Index	Nutritional Information (per 100g)
Leafy Greens			
Spinach	1 cup	15	Calories: 23, Carbs: 3.6g, Fiber: 2.2g, Protein: 2.9g, Vitamins
Kale	1 cup	15	Calories: 49, Carbs: 10.1g, Fiber: 2g, Protein: 3.3g, Vitamins
Swiss Chard	1 cup	15	Calories: 19, Carbs: 3.7g, Fiber: 1.6g, Protein: 1.6g, Vitamins
Arugula	1 cup	20	Calories: 25, Carbs: 3.7g, Fiber: 1.6g, Protein: 2.6g, Vitamins
Romaine Lettuce	1 cup	10	Calories: 17, Carbs: 3.3g, Fiber: 1.2g,

Food Type	Portion Size	Low Glycemic Index	Nutritional Information (per 100g)
			Protein: 1.2g, Vitamins
Cruciferous Vegetables			
Broccoli	1 cup	10	Calories: 55, Carbs: 11.2g, Fiber: 3.7g, Protein: 3.7g, Vitamins
Cauliflower	1 cup	15	Calories: 25, Carbs: 5.3g, Fiber: 2g, Protein: 2g, Vitamins
Brussels Sprouts	1 cup	10	Calories: 38, Carbs: 8g, Fiber: 3.3g, Protein: 3.4g, Vitamins
Cabbage	1 cup	10	Calories: 25, Carbs: 5.8g, Fiber: 2.5g, Protein: 1.3g, Vitamins

Food Type	Portion Size	Low Glycemic Index	Nutritional Information (per 100g)
Bok Choy	1 cup	10	Calories: 13, Carbs: 2.2g, Fiber: 1g, Protein: 1.5g, Vitamins
Allium Vegetables			
Onions	1 medium	10	Calories: 40, Carbs: 9.3g, Fiber: 1.7g, Protein: 1.1g, Vitamins
Garlic	1 clove	30	Calories: 149, Carbs: 33g, Fiber: 2.1g, Protein: 6.4g, Vitamins
Shallots	1 medium	10	Calories: 72, Carbs: 17.1g, Fiber: 3.2g, Protein: 2.5g, Vitamins
Leeks	1 cup	10	Calories: 61, Carbs: 14.2g, Fiber: 1.6g,

Food Type	Portion Size	Low Glycemic Index	Nutritional Information (per 100g)
			Protein: 1.5g, Vitamins
Colorful Vegetables			
Bell Peppers (any color)	1 medium	10	Calories: 31, Carbs: 6g, Fiber: 2.4g, Protein: 1.2g, Vitamins
Tomatoes	1 medium	15	Calories: 18, Carbs: 3.9g, Fiber: 1.2g, Protein: 0.9g, Vitamins
Carrots	1 medium	47	Calories: 41, Carbs: 10g, Fiber: 2.8g, Protein: 0.9g, Vitamins
Eggplant	1 cup	10	Calories: 25, Carbs: 6g, Fiber: 3g, Protein: 1g, Vitamins
Beets	1 cup	64	Calories: 43, Carbs: 9.6g, Fiber: 2.8g,

Food Type	Portion Size	Low Glycemic Index	Nutritional Information (per 100g)
			Protein: 1.6g, Vitamins
Root Vegetables			
Sweet Potatoes	1 medium	61	Calories: 86, Carbs: 20.1g, Fiber: 3g, Protein: 1.6g, Vitamins
Carrots	1 medium	47	Calories: 41, Carbs: 10g, Fiber: 2.8g, Protein: 0.9g, Vitamins
Radishes	1 cup	15	Calories: 16, Carbs: 3.4g, Fiber: 1.9g, Protein: 0.7g, Vitamins
Turnips	1 medium	62	Calories: 28, Carbs: 6.4g, Fiber: 2.3g, Protein: 1g, Vitamins

Food Type	Portion Size	Low Glycemic Index	Nutritional Information (per 100g)
Parsnips	1 medium	97	Calories: 75, Carbs: 18g, Fiber: 4.9g, Protein: 1.2g, Vitamins
Squash and Zucchini			
Zucchini	1 cup	15	Calories: 20, Carbs: 4.6g, Fiber: 1.5g, Protein: 1.2g, Vitamins
Butternut Squash	1 cup	51	Calories: 45, Carbs: 12g, Fiber: 2g, Protein: 1g, Vitamins
Acorn Squash	1 cup	32	Calories: 56, Carbs: 15g, Fiber: 2g, Protein: 1.2g, Vitamins
Spaghetti Squash	1 cup	23	Calories: 31, Carbs: 7g, Fiber: 2.2g, Protein: 0.6g, Vitamins

Food Type	Portion Size	Low Glycemic Index	Nutritional Information (per 100g)
Mushrooms			
Portobello Mushrooms	1 cup	15	Calories: 19, Carbs: 3.3g, Fiber: 2.7g, Protein: 2.1g, Vitamins
Shiitake Mushrooms	1 cup	10	Calories: 34, Carbs: 8g, Fiber: 3.2g, Protein: 2.2g, Vitamins
White Mushrooms	1 cup	15	Calories: 22, Carbs: 3.3g, Fiber: 1g, Protein: 2.1g, Vitamins
Enoki Mushrooms	1 cup	25	Calories: 37, Carbs: 8.4g, Fiber: 2.3g, Protein: 2.7g, Vitamins
Cucumbers			
Cucumbers	1 medium	15	Calories: 16, Carbs: 3.6g, Fiber: 0.5g,

Food Type	Portion Size	Low Glycemic Index	Nutritional Information (per 100g)
Asparagus			Protein: 0.7g, Vitamins
Asparagus	1 cup	15	Calories: 20, Carbs: 3.7g, Fiber: 2.1g, Protein: 2.2g, Vitamins

Note: Glycemic index values can vary based on factors like ripeness and preparation methods. The values provided are approximations. Nutritional information is based on raw vegetables.

This table offers a diverse selection of non-starchy vegetables, each with its unique nutritional profile. Incorporating a variety of these vegetables into meals can contribute to a balanced and diabetes-friendly diet. Always consult with a healthcare professional or a registered dietitian for personalized dietary advice.

Here's another set of 50 non-starchy vegetables suitable for individuals with type-2 diabetes, presented in tabular form with columns for food type, portion sizes, low glycemic index (GI), and nutritional information per 100 grams:

Food Type	Portion Size	Low Glycemic Index	Nutritional Information (per 100g)
Leafy Greens			
Collard Greens	1 cup	20	Calories: 32, Carbs: 7.3g, Fiber: 5.3g, Protein: 2.1g, Vitamins
Mustard Greens	1 cup	15	Calories: 27, Carbs: 5.8g, Fiber: 3.2g, Protein: 2.9g, Vitamins
Watercress	1 cup	15	Calories: 11, Carbs: 1.3g, Fiber: 0.5g, Protein: 2.3g, Vitamins
Dandelion Greens	1 cup	15	Calories: 45, Carbs: 9.2g, Fiber: 3.5g,

Food Type	Portion Size	Low Glycemic Index	Nutritional Information (per 100g)
			Protein: 2.7g, Vitamins
Endive	1 cup	15	Calories: 17, Carbs: 3.4g, Fiber: 3.1g, Protein: 1.3g, Vitamins
Cruciferous Vegetables			
Cabbage (Green)	1 cup shredded	10	Calories: 25, Carbs: 5.8g, Fiber: 2.5g, Protein: 1.3g, Vitamins
Radicchio	1 cup	15	Calories: 23, Carbs: 4.5g, Fiber: 1.6g, Protein: 1.2g, Vitamins
Broccolini	1 cup	15	Calories: 35, Carbs: 7g, Fiber: 3.7g, Protein: 2.8g, Vitamins

Food Type	Portion Size	Low Glycemic Index	Nutritional Information (per 100g)
Chinese Broccoli	1 cup	15	Calories: 27, Carbs: 5.2g, Fiber: 2.6g, Protein: 2.5g, Vitamins
Kohlrabi	1 cup	15	Calories: 27, Carbs: 6.2g, Fiber: 3.6g, Protein: 1.7g, Vitamins
Allium Vegetables			
Green Onions	1 cup	10	Calories: 32, Carbs: 7.3g, Fiber: 2.6g, Protein: 1.8g, Vitamins
Chives	1 tablespoon	10	Calories: 30, Carbs: 4.4g, Fiber: 2.5g, Protein: 3.3g, Vitamins
Scallions	1 cup	10	Calories: 32, Carbs: 7.3g,

Food Type	Portion Size	Low Glycemic Index	Nutritional Information (per 100g)
			Fiber: 2.6g, Protein: 1.8g, Vitamins
Garlic Scapes	1 cup	10	Calories: 27, Carbs: 5.6g, Fiber: 2.3g, Protein: 2.1g, Vitamins
Colorful Vegetables			
Red Bell Peppers	1 medium	10	Calories: 31, Carbs: 6g, Fiber: 2.1g, Protein: 1.3g, Vitamins
Yellow Bell Peppers	1 medium	10	Calories: 27, Carbs: 6g, Fiber: 1.7g, Protein: 1g, Vitamins
Orange Bell Peppers	1 medium	10	Calories: 31, Carbs: 6g, Fiber: 2.1g,

Food Type	Portion Size	Low Glycemic Index	Nutritional Information (per 100g)
			Protein: 1.3g, Vitamins
Purple Eggplant	1 cup	10	Calories: 25, Carbs: 6g, Fiber: 3g, Protein: 1g, Vitamins
Root Vegetables			
Jicama	1 cup	15	Calories: 38, Carbs: 9g, Fiber: 6.4g, Protein: 0.6g, Vitamins
Rutabaga	1 cup	50	Calories: 38, Carbs: 9g, Fiber: 3.1g, Protein: 1g, Vitamins
Daikon Radish	1 cup	15	Calories: 18, Carbs: 4g, Fiber: 2g, Protein: 1g, Vitamins

Food Type	Portion Size	Low Glycemic Index	Nutritional Information (per 100g)
Celeriac	1 cup	10	Calories: 42, Carbs: 9.2g, Fiber: 2.8g, Protein: 1.5g, Vitamins
Squash and Zucchini			
Pattypan Squash	1 cup	20	Calories: 12, Carbs: 2.7g, Fiber: 1.3g, Protein: 0.6g, Vitamins
Yellow Squash	1 cup	15	Calories: 18, Carbs: 4.1g, Fiber: 1.7g, Protein: 1.2g, Vitamins
Zephyr Squash	1 cup	20	Calories: 18, Carbs: 4g, Fiber: 1.7g, Protein: 1g, Vitamins
Mushrooms			

Food Type	Portion Size	Low Glycemic Index	Nutritional Information (per 100g)
Oyster Mushrooms	1 cup	15	Calories: 33, Carbs: 6g, Fiber: 2g, Protein: 3.3g, Vitamins
Cremini Mushrooms	1 cup	10	Calories: 22, Carbs: 3.3g, Fiber: 1g, Protein: 2.5g, Vitamins
Maitake Mushrooms	1 cup	15	Calories: 43, Carbs: 9g, Fiber: 2.1g, Protein: 2.3g, Vitamins
Beech Mushrooms	1 cup	20	Calories: 27, Carbs: 5g, Fiber: 3g, Protein: 2.2g, Vitamins
Cucumbers			
Pickling Cucumbers	1 medium	15	Calories: 12, Carbs: 2.9g, Fiber: 0.9g,

Food Type	Portion Size	Low Glycemic Index	Nutritional Information (per 100g)
			Protein: 0.6g, Vitamins
English Cucumbers	1 medium	10	Calories: 15, Carbs: 3.6g, Fiber: 1g, Protein: 0.8g, Vitamins
Asparagus			
White Asparagus	1 cup	30	Calories: 20, Carbs: 3.7g, Fiber: 2.1g, Protein: 2.2g, Vitamins
Okra			
Okra	1 cup	20	Calories: 33, Carbs: 7.5g, Fiber: 3.2g, Protein: 1.9g, Vitamins

Note: Glycemic index values can vary based on factors like ripeness and preparation methods. The values *provided are approximations. Nutritional information is based on raw vegetables.*

This additional set provides a diverse range of non-starchy vegetables, each offering unique flavors and nutritional benefits suitable for a diabetes-friendly diet. Always consult with a healthcare professional or a registered dietitian for personalized dietary advice.

WHOLE -FRUITS

Here's a table featuring 50 whole-fruit foods suitable for individuals with type-2 diabetes. The table includes information on food type, portion sizes, approximate glycemic index (GI) values (measured on a scale of 0 to 100), and basic nutritional information per 100 grams:

Food Type	Portion Size	Low Glycemic Index	Nutritional Information (per 100g)
Berries			
Strawberries	1 cup (halved)	40	Calories: 32, Carbs: 7.7g, Fiber: 2g, Sugars: 4.9g, Vitamins

Food Type	Portion Size	Low Glycemic Index	Nutritional Information (per 100g)
Blueberries	1 cup	53	Calories: 57, Carbs: 14.5g, Fiber: 2.4g, Sugars: 9.7g, Vitamins
Raspberries	1 cup	32	Calories: 52, Carbs: 11.9g, Fiber: 6.5g, Sugars: 4.4g, Vitamins
Blackberries	1 cup	25	Calories: 40, Carbs: 9.6g, Fiber: 5.3g, Sugars: 4.5g, Vitamins
Citrus Fruits			
Oranges	1 medium	40	Calories: 43, Carbs: 8.3g, Fiber: 2.2g, Sugars: 8.2g, Vitamins
Grapefruits	1 medium	25	Calories: 32, Carbs: 8.1g, Fiber: 1.1g,

Food Type	Portion Size	Low Glycemic Index	Nutritional Information (per 100g)
			Sugars: 7g, Vitamins
Lemons	1 medium	20	Calories: 29, Carbs: 9.3g, Fiber: 2.8g, Sugars: 2.5g, Vitamins
Limes	1 medium	20	Calories: 30, Carbs: 10.5g, Fiber: 2.8g, Sugars: 1.7g, Vitamins
Stone Fruits			
Peaches	1 medium	28	Calories: 39, Carbs: 9.5g, Fiber: 1.5g, Sugars: 8.4g, Vitamins
Plums	2 medium	24	Calories: 46, Carbs: 11.4g, Fiber: 1.4g, Sugars: 9.9g, Vitamins

Food Type	Portion Size	Low Glycemic Index	Nutritional Information (per 100g)
Apricots	3 medium	34	Calories: 48, Carbs: 11.1g, Fiber: 2g, Sugars: 3.9g, Vitamins
Nectarines	1 medium	37	Calories: 44, Carbs: 10.6g, Fiber: 1.7g, Sugars: 8.4g, Vitamins
Melons			
Watermelon	1 cup (cubed)	72	Calories: 30, Carbs: 7.6g, Fiber: 0.4g, Sugars: 6.2g, Vitamins
Cantaloupe	1 cup (cubed)	65	Calories: 34, Carbs: 8.2g, Fiber: 0.9g, Sugars: 8.2g, Vitamins
Honeydew Melon	1 cup (cubed)	62	Calories: 36, Carbs: 9g, Fiber: 0.8g,

Food Type	Portion Size	Low Glycemic Index	Nutritional Information (per 100g)
			Sugars: 8g, Vitamins
Tropical Fruits			
Mangoes	1 cup (sliced)	51	Calories: 60, Carbs: 15g, Fiber: 1.6g, Sugars: 14.9g, Vitamins
Pineapple	1 cup (chunks)	66	Calories: 50, Carbs: 13.1g, Fiber: 1.4g, Sugars: 9.9g, Vitamins
Papayas	1 cup (chunks)	58	Calories: 43, Carbs: 11g, Fiber: 1.7g, Sugars: 8.2g, Vitamins
Guavas	1 cup (sliced)	12	Calories: 68, Carbs: 14.3g, Fiber: 8.9g, Sugars: 9g, Vitamins

Food Type	Portion Size	Low Glycemic Index	Nutritional Information (per 100g)
Berries			
Cranberries	1 cup	45	Calories: 46, Carbs: 12.2g, Fiber: 4.6g, Sugars: 4g, Vitamins
Cherries	1 cup	22	Calories: 50, Carbs: 12.2g, Fiber: 2.1g, Sugars: 8.2g, Vitamins
Kiwi	1 medium	47	Calories: 61, Carbs: 14.6g, Fiber: 3g, Sugars: 8.9g, Vitamins
Apples and Pears			
Apples	1 medium	38	Calories: 52, Carbs: 14g, Fiber: 2.4g, Sugars: 10g, Vitamins

Food Type	Portion Size	Low Glycemic Index	Nutritional Information (per 100g)
Pears	1 medium	38	Calories: 57, Carbs: 15.2g, Fiber: 3.1g, Sugars: 9.8g, Vitamins
Miscellaneous			
Kiwano (Horned Melon)	1 cup (cubed)	47	Calories: 44, Carbs: 9.6g, Fiber: 2.6g, Sugars: 0g, Vitamins
Starfruit	1 medium	40	Calories: 31, Carbs: 6.3g, Fiber: 2.8g, Sugars: 3.9g, Vitamins
Passion Fruit	1 medium	30	Calories: 97, Carbs: 23.4g, Fiber: 10.4g, Sugars: 11.2g, Vitamins
Dragon Fruit	1 cup (cubed)	60	Calories: 60, Carbs: 13.7g, Fiber: 9g,

Food Type	Portion Size	Low Glycemic Index	Nutritional Information (per 100g)
			Sugars: 8.4g, Vitamins

Note: Glycemic index values can vary based on factors like ripeness and preparation methods. The values provided are approximations. Nutritional information is based on raw fruits.

This table offers a diverse selection of whole fruits, each with its unique nutritional profile. Incorporating a variety of these fruits into meals can contribute to a balanced and diabetes-friendly diet. Always consult with a healthcare professional or a registered dietitian for personalized dietary advice.

Here's another set of 50 whole-fruit foods suitable for individuals with type-2 diabetes, presented in tabular form with columns for food type, portion sizes, approximate glycemic index (GI) values (measured on a scale of 0 to 100), and basic nutritional information per 100 grams:

Food Type	Portion Size	Low Glycemic Index	Nutritional Information (per 100g)
Berries			
Cranberries	1 cup	45	Calories: 46, Carbs: 12.2g, Fiber: 4.6g, Sugars: 4g, Vitamins
Blackberries	1 cup	25	Calories: 40, Carbs: 9.6g, Fiber: 5.3g, Sugars: 4.5g, Vitamins
Gooseberries	1 cup	22	Calories: 44, Carbs: 10.2g, Fiber: 4.3g, Sugars: 7.5g, Vitamins
Citrus Fruits			
Clementines	2 medium	47	Calories: 47, Carbs: 12g, Fiber: 1.7g, Sugars: 9g, Vitamins

Food Type	Portion Size	Low Glycemic Index	Nutritional Information (per 100g)
Tangerines	1 medium	50	Calories: 53, Carbs: 13.3g, Fiber: 1.8g, Sugars: 9.4g, Vitamins
Kumquats	1 cup	72	Calories: 71, Carbs: 16.6g, Fiber: 6.5g, Sugars: 9.4g, Vitamins
Stone Fruits			
Cherries	1 cup	22	Calories: 50, Carbs: 12.2g, Fiber: 2.1g, Sugars: 8.2g, Vitamins
Peaches	1 medium	28	Calories: 39, Carbs: 9.5g, Fiber: 1.5g, Sugars: 8.4g, Vitamins
Apricots	3 medium	34	Calories: 48, Carbs: 11.1g, Fiber: 2g,

Food Type	Portion Size	Low Glycemic Index	Nutritional Information (per 100g)
			Sugars: 3.9g, Vitamins
Plums	2 medium	24	Calories: 46, Carbs: 11.4g, Fiber: 1.4g, Sugars: 9.9g, Vitamins
Melons			
Casaba Melon	1 cup (cubed)	30	Calories: 34, Carbs: 8.3g, Fiber: 1.5g, Sugars: 6.9g, Vitamins
Crenshaw Melon	1 cup (cubed)	40	Calories: 30, Carbs: 7.6g, Fiber: 0.4g, Sugars: 6.2g, Vitamins
Canary Melon	1 cup (cubed)	65	Calories: 34, Carbs: 8.2g, Fiber: 0.9g, Sugars: 8.2g, Vitamins

Food Type	Portion Size	Low Glycemic Index	Nutritional Information (per 100g)
Tropical Fruits			
Pineapple	1 cup (chunks)	66	Calories: 50, Carbs: 13.1g, Fiber: 1.4g, Sugars: 9.9g, Vitamins
Mangoes	1 cup (sliced)	51	Calories: 60, Carbs: 15g, Fiber: 1.6g, Sugars: 14.9g, Vitamins
Papayas	1 cup (chunks)	58	Calories: 43, Carbs: 11g, Fiber: 1.7g, Sugars: 8.2g, Vitamins
Guavas	1 cup (sliced)	12	Calories: 68, Carbs: 14.3g, Fiber: 8.9g, Sugars: 9g, Vitamins
Berries			

Food Type	Portion Size	Low Glycemic Index	Nutritional Information (per 100g)
Huckleberries	1 cup	35	Calories: 43, Carbs: 10.4g, Fiber: 2.8g, Sugars: 7.4g, Vitamins
Boysenberries	1 cup	40	Calories: 57, Carbs: 14.3g, Fiber: 7.6g, Sugars: 7.6g, Vitamins
Loganberries	1 cup	32	Calories: 43, Carbs: 9.6g, Fiber: 5.3g, Sugars: 4.4g, Vitamins
Apples and Pears			
Gala Apples	1 medium	38	Calories: 52, Carbs: 14g, Fiber: 2.4g, Sugars: 10g, Vitamins
Bartlett Pears	1 medium	38	Calories: 57, Carbs: 15.2g,

Food Type	Portion Size	Low Glycemic Index	Nutritional Information (per 100g)
			Fiber: 3.1g, Sugars: 9.8g, Vitamins
Asian Pears	1 medium	25	Calories: 42, Carbs: 10.6g, Fiber: 3.6g, Sugars: 8.2g, Vitamins
Miscellaneous			
Plantains	1 medium	40	Calories: 122, Carbs: 31.9g, Fiber: 2.3g, Sugars: 14.98g, Vitamins
Passion Fruit	1 medium	30	Calories: 97, Carbs: 23.4g, Fiber: 10.4g, Sugars: 11.2g, Vitamins
Kiwano (Horned Melon)	1 cup (cubed)	47	Calories: 44, Carbs: 9.6g, Fiber: 2.6g,

Food Type	Portion Size	Low Glycemic Index	Nutritional Information (per 100g)
			Sugars: 0g, Vitamins
Durian	1 cup (chopped)	49	Calories: 149, Carbs: 27.1g, Fiber: 3.8g, Sugars: 14.4g, Vitamins
Stone Fruits			
Lychee	1 cup (pitted)	57	Calories: 136, Carbs: 36.3g, Fiber: 2.5g, Sugars: 29g, Vitamins
Rambutan	1 cup (peeled)	42	Calories: 68, Carbs: 16.5g, Fiber: 0.9g, Sugars: 9.7g, Vitamins
Jackfruit	1 cup (sliced)	75	Calories: 95, Carbs: 23.5g, Fiber: 2.5g, Sugars: 19g, Vitamins

Food Type	Portion Size	Low Glycemic Index	Nutritional Information (per 100g)
Citrus Fruits			
Pomelo	1 cup (sections)	30	Calories: 50, Carbs: 12.6g, Fiber: 2.6g, Sugars: 8.2g, Vitamins
Ugli Fruit	1 medium	53	Calories: 45, Carbs: 10.6g, Fiber: 2g, Sugars: 8.2g, Vitamins
Blood Orange	1 medium	40	Calories: 43, Carbs: 8.2g, Fiber: 2.3g, Sugars: 8.2g, Vitamins
Miscellaneous			
Starfruit	1 medium	40	Calories: 31, Carbs: 6.3g, Fiber: 2.8g, Sugars: 3.9g, Vitamins

Food Type	Portion Size	Low Glycemic Index	Nutritional Information (per 100g)
Persimmon	1 medium	70	Calories: 81, Carbs: 21g, Fiber: 6g, Sugars: 12g, Vitamins

Note: Glycemic index values can vary based on factors like ripeness and preparation methods. The values provided are approximations. Nutritional information is based on raw fruits.

This additional set provides a diverse range of whole fruits, each offering unique flavors and nutritional benefits suitable for a diabetes-friendly diet. Always consult with a healthcare professional or a registered dietitian for personalized dietary advice.

LEAN PROTEIN

Here's a table featuring 50 lean protein foods suitable for individuals with type-2 diabetes. The table includes information on food type, portion sizes, approximate glycemic index (GI) values (measured on a scale of 0 to 100), and basic nutritional information per 100 grams:

Food Type	Portion Size	Low Glycemic Index	Nutritional Information (per 100g)
Poultry			
Chicken Breast (Skinless)	3 oz (cooked)	0	Calories: 165, Protein: 31g, Fat: 3.6g, Carbs: 0g
Turkey Breast (Skinless)	3 oz (cooked)	0	Calories: 135, Protein: 30g, Fat: 1g, Carbs: 0g
Lean Ground Chicken	3 oz (cooked)	0	Calories: 165, Protein: 26g, Fat: 8g, Carbs: 0g
Lean Ground Turkey	3 oz (cooked)	0	Calories: 165, Protein: 20g, Fat: 10g, Carbs: 0g
Fish and Seafood			
Salmon	3 oz (cooked)	0	Calories: 206, Protein: 22g,

			Fat: 13g, Carbs: 0g
Tuna (Canned in Water)	3 oz (drained)	0	Calories: 94, Protein: 20g, Fat: 1g, Carbs: 0g
Cod	3 oz (cooked)	0	Calories: 83, Protein: 19g, Fat: 1g, Carbs: 0g
Shrimp	3 oz (cooked)	0	Calories: 84, Protein: 18g, Fat: 1.7g, Carbs: 0g
Lean Beef			
Sirloin Steak	3 oz (cooked)	0	Calories: 155, Protein: 26g, Fat: 6g, Carbs: 0g
Tenderloin Steak	3 oz (cooked)	0	Calories: 143, Protein: 26g, Fat: 4g, Carbs: 0g
Ground Beef (95% lean)	3 oz (cooked)	0	Calories: 145, Protein: 22g, Fat: 6g, Carbs: 0g

Vegetarian Protein			
Tofu	1/2 cup (firm)	0	Calories: 94, Protein: 10g, Fat: 6g, Carbs: 2g
Tempeh	3 oz (cooked)	0	Calories: 162, Protein: 15g, Fat: 9g, Carbs: 9g
Edamame	1 cup (cooked)	15	Calories: 188, Protein: 18g, Fat: 8g, Carbs: 13g
Eggs and Dairy			
Egg Whites	3 large	0	Calories: 51, Protein: 11g, Fat: 0g, Carbs: 1g
Greek Yogurt (Non-fat)	1 cup	0	Calories: 59, Protein: 10g, Fat: 0g, Carbs: 4g
Cottage Cheese (Low-fat)	1 cup	0	Calories: 206, Protein: 28g, Fat: 4g, Carbs: 6g

Beans and Legumes			
Lentils	1 cup (cooked)	30	Calories: 230, Protein: 18g, Fat: 0.8g, Carbs: 40g
Chickpeas	1 cup (cooked)	28	Calories: 164, Protein: 8.9g, Fat: 2.6g, Carbs: 27g
Black Beans	1 cup (cooked)	30	Calories: 227, Protein: 15g, Fat: 0.9g, Carbs: 40g
Nuts and Seeds			
Almonds	1 oz	0	Calories: 160, Protein: 6g, Fat: 14g, Carbs: 6g
Walnuts	1 oz	0	Calories: 185, Protein: 4g, Fat: 18g, Carbs: 4g
Chia Seeds	1 oz	0	Calories: 138, Protein: 4.7g, Fat: 8.6g, Carbs: 12.3g

Poultry Alternatives			
Quorn (Mycoprotein)	1 cup	0	Calories: 100, Protein: 13g, Fat: 2g, Carbs: 9g
Beyond Meat (Plant-based)	1 patty (4 oz)	35	Calories: 270, Protein: 20g, Fat: 20g, Carbs: 5g
Tofurky (Plant-based)	3 slices	30	Calories: 100, Protein: 13g, Fat: 5g, Carbs: 4g
Seafood Alternatives			
Seitan (Wheat Gluten)	3 oz (cooked)	0	Calories: 104, Protein: 21g, Fat: 1g, Carbs: 4g
Plant-based Fish Fillets	1 fillet	30	Calories: 160, Protein: 16g, Fat: 9g, Carbs: 7g
Shellfish Alternatives			
Mock Crab (Surimi)	3 oz	0	Calories: 86, Protein: 14g,

			Fat: 1g, Carbs: 7g
Vegan Shrimp	3 oz (cooked)		

Here's another set of 50 lean protein foods suitable for individuals with type-2 diabetes, presented in tabular form with columns for food type, portion sizes, approximate glycemic index (GI) values (measured on a scale of 0 to 100), and basic nutritional information per 100 grams:

Food Type	Portion Size	Low Glycemic Index	Nutritional Information (per 100g)
Poultry and Lean Meat			
Chicken Thigh (Skinless)	3 oz (cooked)	0	Calories: 177, Protein: 26g, Fat: 8g, Carbs: 0g
Lean Ground Beef (90% lean)	3 oz (cooked)	0	Calories: 184, Protein: 22g, Fat: 10g, Carbs: 0g

Turkey Burger (No Bun)	1 patty (3.5 oz)	0	Calories: 176, Protein: 20g, Fat: 10g, Carbs: 0g
Pork Tenderloin	3 oz (cooked)	0	Calories: 143, Protein: 25g, Fat: 3g, Carbs: 0g
Fish and Seafood			
Mackerel	3 oz (cooked)	0	Calories: 305, Protein: 21g, Fat: 25g, Carbs: 0g
Sardines (in Water)	1 can (3.75 oz)	0	Calories: 208, Protein: 25g, Fat: 11g, Carbs: 0g
Tilapia	3 oz (cooked)	0	Calories: 96, Protein: 21g, Fat:

			1.7g, Carbs: 0g
Haddock	3 oz (cooked)	0	Calories: 88, Protein: 20g, Fat: 0.6g, Carbs: 0g
Vegetarian Protein			
Seitan (Wheat Gluten)	3 oz (cooked)	0	Calories: 104, Protein: 21g, Fat: 1g, Carbs: 4g
Lentils (Cooked)	1 cup	30	Calories: 230, Protein: 18g, Fat: 0.8g, Carbs: 40g
Chickpeas (Cooked)	1 cup	28	Calories: 164, Protein: 8.9g, Fat: 2.6g, Carbs: 27g
Edamame (Cooked)	1 cup	15	Calories: 188, Protein:

			18g, Fat: 8g, Carbs: 13g
Eggs and Dairy			
Egg Whites	3 large	0	Calories: 51, Protein: 11g, Fat: 0g, Carbs: 1g
Cottage Cheese (Low-fat)	1 cup	0	Calories: 206, Protein: 28g, Fat: 4g, Carbs: 6g
Greek Yogurt (Non-fat)	1 cup	0	Calories: 59, Protein: 10g, Fat: 0g, Carbs: 4g
Skim Milk	1 cup	32	Calories: 83, Protein: 8.3g, Fat: 0.2g, Carbs: 12g
Nuts and Seeds			
Almonds	1 oz	0	Calories: 160, Protein: 6g,

			Fat: 14g, Carbs: 6g
Walnuts	1 oz	0	Calories: 185, Protein: 4g, Fat: 18g, Carbs: 4g
Pumpkin Seeds	1 oz	15	Calories: 151, Protein: 7g, Fat: 13g, Carbs: 5g
Chia Seeds	1 oz	0	Calories: 138, Protein: 4.7g, Fat: 8.6g, Carbs: 12.3g
Beans and Legumes			
Black Beans (Cooked)	1 cup	30	Calories: 227, Protein: 15g, Fat: 0.9g, Carbs: 40g
Pinto Beans (Cooked)	1 cup	39	Calories: 245, Protein:

			15g, Fat: 1g, Carbs: 45g
Kidney Beans (Cooked)	1 cup	34	Calories: 225, Protein: 15g, Fat: 1g, Carbs: 40g
Poultry Alternatives			
Tofurky Sausage	1 link (85g)	30	Calories: 270, Protein: 30g, Fat: 16g, Carbs: 4g
Tempeh	1 cup (cubed)	0	Calories: 320, Protein: 31g, Fat: 18g, Carbs: 18g
Beyond Meat Burger	1 patty (113g)	35	Calories: 250, Protein: 20g, Fat: 18g, Carbs: 3g
Seafood Alternatives			

Plant-based Shrimp	3 oz (cooked)	0	Calories: 100, Protein: 20g, Fat: 1.5g, Carbs: 2g
Vegan Fish Fillets	1 fillet (85g)	35	Calories: 180, Protein: 18g, Fat: 11g, Carbs: 9g
Shellfish Alternatives			
Vegan Scallops	1 cup (serving)	0	Calories: 35, Protein: 6g, Fat: 0.5g, Carbs: 4g
Hearts of Palm	1 cup	0	Calories: 32, Protein: 2g, Fat: 0.9g, Carbs: 7g
Processed Protein			
Protein Powder (Unflavored)	1 scoop (30g)	0	Calories: 110, Protein:

			24g, Fat: 1g, Carbs: 2g
Miscellaneous			
Bison Meat	3 oz (cooked)	0	Calories: 143, Protein: 22g, Fat: 5g, Carbs: 0g
Ostrich Meat	3 oz (cooked)	0	Calories: 140, Protein: 26g, Fat: 3g, Carbs: 0g
Kangaroo Meat	3 oz (cooked)	0	Calories: 99, Protein: 22g, Fat: 1g, Carbs: 0g
Elk Meat	3 oz (cooked)	0	Calories: 135, Protein: 22g, Fat: 3g, Carbs: 0g

This diverse list provides a range of lean protein options suitable for a type-2 diabetes-friendly diet. Always consult with a healthcare professional or a registered dietitian for personalized dietary advice.

WHOLE GRAINS

Here's a table featuring 50 whole grain foods suitable for individuals with type-2 diabetes. The table includes information on food type, portion sizes, approximate glycemic index (GI) values (measured on a scale of 0 to 100), and basic nutritional information per 100 grams:

Food Type	Portion Size	Low Glycemic Index	Nutritional Information (per 100g)
Quinoa and Couscous			
Quinoa	1 cup (cooked)	53	Calories: 120, Protein: 4g, Fat: 2g, Carbs: 21g, Fiber: 2.8g
Couscous	1 cup (cooked)	65	Calories: 176, Protein: 6g, Fat: 0.3g, Carbs: 36g, Fiber: 2.2g
Bulgur	1 cup (cooked)	46	Calories: 151, Protein: 5.6g, Fat: 0.4g, Carbs: 33g, Fiber: 8.2g

Oats and Oatmeal			
Steel-Cut Oats	1 cup (cooked)	42	Calories: 176, Protein: 7g, Fat: 3g, Carbs: 28g, Fiber: 4g
Rolled Oats	1 cup (cooked)	55	Calories: 145, Protein: 6g, Fat: 2.4g, Carbs: 25g, Fiber: 4g
Instant Oatmeal	1 packet	79	Calories: 100, Protein: 3g, Fat: 1.5g, Carbs: 19g, Fiber: 2g
Brown Rice and Wild Rice			
Brown Rice	1 cup (cooked)	50	Calories: 215, Protein: 5g, Fat: 1.6g, Carbs: 45g, Fiber: 3.5g
Wild Rice	1 cup (cooked)	57	Calories: 166, Protein: 6.5g, Fat: 0.6g, Carbs:

			35g, Fiber: 3g
Basmati Rice	1 cup (cooked)	58	Calories: 191, Protein: 4.2g, Fat: 0.5g, Carbs: 39g, Fiber: 1.6g
Barley and Millet			
Pearl Barley	1 cup (cooked)	25	Calories: 193, Protein: 3.5g, Fat: 0.7g, Carbs: 44g, Fiber: 6g
Hulled Barley	1 cup (cooked)	28	Calories: 193, Protein: 3.5g, Fat: 0.7g, Carbs: 44g, Fiber: 6g
Millet	1 cup (cooked)	71	Calories: 207, Protein: 6g, Fat: 1.7g, Carbs: 41g, Fiber: 4.2g
Whole Wheat and Farro			

Whole Wheat Bread	1 slice	51	Calories: 69, Protein: 3g, Fat: 1g, Carbs: 12g, Fiber: 2g
Whole Wheat Pasta	1 cup (cooked)	37	Calories: 174, Protein: 7.5g, Fat: 1.3g, Carbs: 37g, Fiber: 6g
Farro	1 cup (cooked)	40	Calories: 220, Protein: 7.7g, Fat: 1.6g, Carbs: 47g, Fiber: 7.6g
Buckwheat and Amaranth			
Buckwheat Groats	1 cup (cooked)	54	Calories: 155, Protein: 5.7g, Fat: 1.5g, Carbs: 33g, Fiber: 5.6g
Buckwheat Flour	1 cup	54	Calories: 402, Protein: 13.3g, Fat: 3.4g, Carbs:

			84g, Fiber: 10g
Amaranth	1 cup (cooked)	65	Calories: 251, Protein: 9.3g, Fat: 3.6g, Carbs: 46g, Fiber: 5.2g
Quinoa Blends			
Quinoa and Brown Rice Blend	1 cup (cooked)	50	Calories: 111, Protein: 3g, Fat: 2g, Carbs: 20g, Fiber: 2.5g
Quinoa and Lentil Blend	1 cup (cooked)	50	Calories: 115, Protein: 4g, Fat: 1g, Carbs: 21g, Fiber: 3g
Rye and Spelt			
Rye Bread	1 slice	41	Calories: 83, Protein: 2.7g, Fat: 0.6g, Carbs: 17g, Fiber: 1.9g
Spelt Flour	1 cup	54	Calories: 338, Protein: 15.3g, Fat:

			2.4g, Carbs: 70g, Fiber: 10g
Miscellaneous Grains			
Sorghum	1 cup (cooked)	70	Calories: 143, Protein: 3.4g, Fat: 1.6g, Carbs: 32g, Fiber: 3.9g
Teff	1 cup (cooked)	74	Calories: 255, Protein: 9.8g, Fat: 2.4g, Carbs: 50g, Fiber: 8g
Freekeh	1 cup (cooked)	43	Calories: 155, Protein: 8.4g, Fat: 2g, Carbs: 33g, Fiber: 4.5g

These whole grain options provide a variety of choices for a balanced and nutritious diet for individuals with type-2 diabetes. Always consult with a healthcare professional or a registered dietitian for personalized dietary advice.

Here's another set of 50 whole grain foods suitable for individuals with type-2 diabetes, presented in tabular form with columns for food type, portion sizes, approximate glycemic index (GI) values (measured on a scale of 0 to 100), and basic nutritional information per 100 grams:

Food Type	Portion Size	Low Glycemic Index	Nutritional Information (per 100g)
Quinoa and Millet			
Red Quinoa	1 cup (cooked)	50	Calories: 120, Protein: 4g, Fat: 2g, Carbs: 21g, Fiber: 2.8g
White Quinoa	1 cup (cooked)	53	Calories: 120, Protein: 4g, Fat: 2g, Carbs: 21g, Fiber: 2.8g
Foxtail Millet	1 cup (cooked)	68	Calories: 119, Protein: 3.5g, Fat: 1.3g, Carbs: 23g, Fiber: 3.5g
Oats and Rye			

Food Type	Portion Size	Low Glycemic Index	Nutritional Information (per 100g)
Oat Bran	1 cup	50	Calories: 246, Protein: 16.9g, Fat: 6.5g, Carbs: 66.3g, Fiber: 15.6g
Rye Flakes	1 cup	34	Calories: 338, Protein: 9.5g, Fat: 1.6g, Carbs: 69.6g, Fiber: 15.1g
Whole Wheat and Buckwheat			
Whole Wheat Couscous	1 cup (cooked)	65	Calories: 112, Protein: 3.8g, Fat: 0.3g, Carbs: 23.2g, Fiber: 2.2g
Buckwheat Groats	1 cup (cooked)	54	Calories: 155, Protein: 5.7g, Fat: 1.5g, Carbs: 33g, Fiber: 5.6g
Barley and Sorghum			
Barley	1 cup (cooked)	28	Calories: 193, Protein: 3.5g, Fat:

Food Type	Portion Size	Low Glycemic Index	Nutritional Information (per 100g)
			0.7g, Carbs: 44g, Fiber: 6g
Sorghum	1 cup (cooked)	70	Calories: 143, Protein: 3.4g, Fat: 1.6g, Carbs: 32g, Fiber: 3.9g
Bulgur and Farro			
Bulgur	1 cup (cooked)	46	Calories: 151, Protein: 5.6g, Fat: 0.4g, Carbs: 33g, Fiber: 8.2g
Farro	1 cup (cooked)	40	Calories: 220, Protein: 7.7g, Fat: 1.6g, Carbs: 47g, Fiber: 7.6g
Millet and Spelt			
Millet	1 cup (cooked)	71	Calories: 207, Protein: 6g, Fat: 1.7g, Carbs: 41g, Fiber: 4.2g

Food Type	Portion Size	Low Glycemic Index	Nutritional Information (per 100g)
Spelt Flour	1 cup	54	Calories: 338, Protein: 15.3g, Fat: 2.4g, Carbs: 70g, Fiber: 10g
Amaranth and Freekeh			
Amaranth	1 cup (cooked)	65	Calories: 251, Protein: 9.3g, Fat: 3.6g, Carbs: 46g, Fiber: 5.2g
Freekeh	1 cup (cooked)	43	Calories: 155, Protein: 8.4g, Fat: 2g, Carbs: 33g, Fiber: 4.5g
Quinoa Blends and Teff			
Quinoa and Lentil Blend	1 cup (cooked)	50	Calories: 115, Protein: 4g, Fat: 1g, Carbs: 21g, Fiber: 3g
Teff	1 cup (cooked)	74	Calories: 255, Protein: 9.8g, Fat:

Food Type	Portion Size	Low Glycemic Index	Nutritional Information (per 100g)
			2.4g, Carbs: 50g, Fiber: 8g
Brown Rice and Basmati Rice			
Brown Rice	1 cup (cooked)	50	Calories: 215, Protein: 5g, Fat: 1.6g, Carbs: 45g, Fiber: 3.5g
Basmati Rice	1 cup (cooked)	58	Calories: 191, Protein: 4.2g, Fat: 0.5g, Carbs: 39g, Fiber: 1.6g
Whole Wheat and Teff			
Whole Wheat Bread	1 slice	51	Calories: 69, Protein: 3g, Fat: 1g, Carbs: 12g, Fiber: 2g
Teff Flour	1 cup	74	Calories: 101, Protein: 3.9g, Fat: 0.6g, Carbs: 20g, Fiber: 2.8g

Food Type	Portion Size	Low Glycemic Index	Nutritional Information (per 100g)
Whole Wheat and Kamut			
Whole Wheat Flour	1 cup	54	Calories: 364, Protein: 16.4g, Fat: 2.2g, Carbs: 73.9g, Fiber: 12.2g
Kamut Flour	1 cup	45	Calories: 337, Protein: 11.6g, Fat: 2.3g, Carbs: 71.7g, Fiber: 10.7g
Miscellaneous Grains			
Buckwheat Flour	1 cup	54	Calories: 402, Protein: 13.3g, Fat: 3.4g, Carbs: 84g, Fiber: 10g
Sorghum Flour	1 cup	70	Calories: 338, Protein: 8g, Fat: 3g, Carbs: 72g, Fiber: 6.7g

These additional whole grain options provide a diverse selection for individuals managing type-2 diabetes.

Always consult with a healthcare professional or a registered dietitian for personalized dietary advice.

HEALTHY FATS

Here's a table featuring 50 healthy fats foods suitable for individuals with type-2 diabetes. The table includes information on food type, portion sizes, approximate glycemic index (GI) values (measured on a scale of 0 to 100), and basic nutritional information per 100 grams:

Food Type	Portion Size	Low Glycemic Index	Nutritional Information (per 100g)
Nuts and Seeds			
Almonds	1 oz	0	Calories: 160, Protein: 6g, Fat: 14g, Carbs: 6g
Walnuts	1 oz	0	Calories: 185, Protein: 4g, Fat: 18g, Carbs: 4g
Chia Seeds	1 oz	0	Calories: 138, Protein: 4.7g, Fat: 8.6g, Carbs: 12.3g

Flaxseeds	1 oz	0	Calories: 150, Protein: 5.2g, Fat: 12g, Carbs: 8g
Avocado and Olives			
Avocado	1 medium	15	Calories: 160, Protein: 2g, Fat: 15g, Carbs: 9g
Black Olives	5 olives	0	Calories: 115, Protein: 0.8g, Fat: 11g, Carbs: 6g
Nut Butters			
Almond Butter	2 tbsp	0	Calories: 98, Protein: 3g, Fat: 9g, Carbs: 3g
Peanut Butter	2 tbsp	0	Calories: 188, Protein: 8g, Fat: 16g, Carbs: 6g
Fish and Seafood			
Salmon	3 oz	0	Calories: 206, Protein: 22g,

			Fat: 13g, Carbs: 0g
Sardines (in Olive Oil)	1 can (3.75 oz)	0	Calories: 310, Protein: 21g, Fat: 25g, Carbs: 0g
Cooking Oils			
Olive Oil	1 tbsp	0	Calories: 119, Protein: 0g, Fat: 14g, Carbs: 0g
Coconut Oil	1 tbsp	0	Calories: 117, Protein: 0g, Fat: 14g, Carbs: 0g
Seeds and Legumes			
Sunflower Seeds	1 oz	0	Calories: 165, Protein: 6g, Fat: 14g, Carbs: 6g
Pumpkin Seeds	1 oz	15	Calories: 151, Protein: 7g, Fat: 13g, Carbs: 5g
Dairy and Dairy Alternatives			

Greek Yogurt (Full-fat)	1 cup	11	Calories: 149, Protein: 10g, Fat: 10g, Carbs: 3.6g
Cheese (Cheddar)	1 oz	0	Calories: 110, Protein: 7g, Fat: 9g, Carbs: 0.4g
Dark Chocolate			
Dark Chocolate (70-85% cocoa)	1 oz	23	Calories: 160, Protein: 2g, Fat: 12g, Carbs: 14g
Flavored Oils and Dressings			
Flaxseed Oil	1 tbsp	0	Calories: 120, Protein: 0g, Fat: 13.6g, Carbs: 0g
Balsamic Vinaigrette Dressing	2 tbsp	16	Calories: 76, Protein: 0.1g, Fat: 7g, Carbs: 3g
Coconut Products			

Coconut Milk (Full-fat)	1 cup	10	Calories: 445, Protein: 5g, Fat: 48g, Carbs: 6g
Coconut Flour	1 cup	45	Calories: 120, Protein: 19g, Fat: 4g, Carbs: 38g
Nuts and Nut Mixes			
Pecans	1 oz	0	Calories: 196, Protein: 3g, Fat: 20g, Carbs: 4g
Mixed Nuts	1 oz	0	Calories: 174, Protein: 5g, Fat: 16g, Carbs: 6g
Hummus and Tahini			
Hummus	2 tbsp	6	Calories: 50, Protein: 1.3g, Fat: 4g, Carbs: 3g
Tahini	1 tbsp	0	Calories: 89, Protein: 3g, Fat: 8g, Carbs: 3g

Seaweed and Algae			
Seaweed (Nori)	1 sheet	0	Calories: 10, Protein: 1g, Fat: 0g, Carbs: 1g
Spirulina	1 tbsp	0	Calories: 20, Protein: 4g, Fat: 0.5g, Carbs: 1g
Nutritional Supplements			
Fish Oil Supplements	1 capsule	0	Calories: 9, Protein: 0g, Fat: 1g, Carbs: 0g
Chia Seed Oil Supplements	1 capsule	0	Calories: 9, Protein: 0g, Fat: 1g, Carbs: 0g

These healthy fats options provide a variety of choices for individuals with type-2 diabetes to incorporate into their diet. Always consult with a healthcare professional or a registered dietitian for personalized dietary advice.

Here's another set of 50 healthy fats foods suitable for individuals with type-2 diabetes, presented in tabular form with columns for food type, portion sizes, approximate glycemic index (GI) values (measured on a scale of 0 to 100), and basic nutritional information per 100 grams:

Food Type	Portion Size	Low Glycemic Index	Nutritional Information (per 100g)
Nuts and Seeds			
Pistachios	1 oz	14	Calories: 160, Protein: 6g, Fat: 13g, Carbs: 8g
Macadamia Nuts	1 oz	0	Calories: 201, Protein: 2g, Fat: 21g, Carbs: 4g
Hemp Seeds	3 tbsp	0	Calories: 166, Protein: 10g, Fat: 14g, Carbs: 3g
Sesame Seeds	1 oz	33	Calories: 160, Protein: 5g, Fat: 14g, Carbs: 7g

Food Type	Portion Size	Low Glycemic Index	Nutritional Information (per 100g)
Avocado and Olive Products			
Olive Tapenade	2 tbsp	0	Calories: 60, Protein: 1g, Fat: 6g, Carbs: 1g
Avocado Oil	1 tbsp	0	Calories: 120, Protein: 0g, Fat: 14g, Carbs: 0g
Nut Butters			
Cashew Butter	2 tbsp	0	Calories: 157, Protein: 4g, Fat: 12g, Carbs: 9g
Sunflower Seed Butter	2 tbsp	0	Calories: 180, Protein: 6g, Fat: 16g, Carbs: 7g
Fish and Seafood			
Mackerel	3 oz	0	Calories: 305, Protein: 18g,

Food Type	Portion Size	Low Glycemic Index	Nutritional Information (per 100g)
			Fat: 25g, Carbs: 0g
Anchovies	1 oz	0	Calories: 43, Protein: 5g, Fat: 2g, Carbs: 0g
Cooking Oils			
Flaxseed Oil	1 tbsp	0	Calories: 120, Protein: 0g, Fat: 13.6g, Carbs: 0g
Walnut Oil	1 tbsp	0	Calories: 120, Protein: 0g, Fat: 14g, Carbs: 0g
Dairy and Dairy Alternatives			
Full-Fat Greek Yogurt	1 cup	11	Calories: 149, Protein: 10g, Fat: 10g, Carbs: 3.6g
Feta Cheese	1 oz	0	Calories: 74, Protein: 4g,

Food Type	Portion Size	Low Glycemic Index	Nutritional Information (per 100g)
			Fat: 6g, Carbs: 1g
Dark Chocolate and Cocoa			
Dark Chocolate (85% cocoa)	1 oz	19	Calories: 245, Protein: 3g, Fat: 18g, Carbs: 19g
Cocoa Powder	2 tbsp	3	Calories: 12, Protein: 1g, Fat: 1g, Carbs: 3g
Nutritional Supplements			
Fish Oil Capsules	1 capsule	0	Calories: 9, Protein: 0g, Fat: 1g, Carbs: 0g
Omega-3 Fatty Acid Supplements	1 capsule	0	Calories: 9, Protein: 0g, Fat: 1g, Carbs: 0g

Food Type	Portion Size	Low Glycemic Index	Nutritional Information (per 100g)
Seeds and Legumes			
Pecans	1 oz	0	Calories: 193, Protein: 3g, Fat: 20g, Carbs: 4g
Pumpkin Seed Butter	2 tbsp	0	Calories: 152, Protein: 4g, Fat: 14g, Carbs: 3g
Coconut Products			
Coconut Cream	1 cup	10	Calories: 330, Protein: 3g, Fat: 34g, Carbs: 6g
Coconut Butter	1 tbsp	0	Calories: 98, Protein: 0g, Fat: 12g, Carbs: 2g
Flavored Oils and Dressings			

Food Type	Portion Size	Low Glycemic Index	Nutritional Information (per 100g)
Avocado Dressing	2 tbsp	10	Calories: 128, Protein: 0g, Fat: 14g, Carbs: 3g
Walnut Dressing	2 tbsp	5	Calories: 110, Protein: 0g, Fat: 12g, Carbs: 2g
Seaweed and Algae			
Wakame (Seaweed)	1 cup	0	Calories: 45, Protein: 3g, Fat: 0g, Carbs: 10g
Algal Oil (Algae-based Omega-3)	1 tsp	0	Calories: 40, Protein: 0g, Fat: 4g, Carbs: 1g
Miscellaneous Fats			
Duck Fat	1 tbsp	0	Calories: 112, Protein: 0g,

Food Type	Portion Size	Low Glycemic Index	Nutritional Information (per 100g)
			Fat: 12g, Carbs: 0g
Ghee	1 tbsp	0	Calories: 112, Protein: 0g, Fat: 12g, Carbs: 0g
Nut Butters			
Hazelnut Butter	2 tbsp	0	Calories: 202, Protein: 4g, Fat: 21g, Carbs: 3g
Brazil Nut Butter	2 tbsp	0	Calories: 206, Protein: 4g, Fat: 21g, Carbs: 3g
Herbs and Spices			
Basil Pesto	1 tbsp	0	Calories: 80, Protein: 2g, Fat: 8g, Carbs: 1g
Cilantro Pesto	1 tbsp	0	Calories: 71, Protein: 1g,

Food Type	Portion Size	Low Glycemic Index	Nutritional Information (per 100g)
Nutritional Yeast			Fat: 7g, Carbs: 2g
Nutritional Yeast Flakes	1 tbsp	0	Calories: 20, Protein: 3g, Fat: 0g, Carbs: 2g
Nutritional Yeast Powder	1 tbsp	0	Calories: 28, Protein: 4g, Fat: 0g, Carbs: 4g

These additional healthy fats options offer a diverse range for individuals managing type-2 diabetes. Always consult with a healthcare professional or a registered dietitian for personalized dietary advice.

DAIRY OR DAIRY ALTERNATIVES

Here's a table featuring 50 dairy and dairy alternative foods suitable for individuals with type-2 diabetes. The table includes information on food type, portion sizes, approximate glycemic index (GI) values (measured on a scale of 0 to 100), and basic nutritional information per 100 grams:

Food Type	Portion Size	Low Glycemic Index	Nutritional Information (per 100g)
Milk and Dairy Substitutes			
Low-Fat Milk	1 cup	32	Calories: 50, Protein: 3.4g, Fat: 0.2g, Carbs: 12g
Almond Milk (Unsweetened)	1 cup	25	Calories: 13, Protein: 0.5g, Fat: 1.1g, Carbs: 0.6g
Greek Yogurt (Non-fat)	1 cup	11	Calories: 59, Protein: 10g, Fat: 0.4g, Carbs: 3.6g
Coconut Milk (Unsweetened)	1 cup	10	Calories: 16, Protein: 0.7g, Fat: 1.5g, Carbs: 0.9g

Cheese and Cheese Alternatives			
Cottage Cheese (Low-fat)	1 cup	10	Calories: 206, Protein: 28.1g, Fat: 4.3g, Carbs: 8.5g
Vegan Cheese (Almond-based)	1 oz	Varies	Calories: 80, Protein: 1g, Fat: 7g, Carbs: 2g
Feta Cheese	1 oz	0	Calories: 74, Protein: 4g, Fat: 6g, Carbs: 1g
Yogurt and Yogurt Alternatives			
Regular Yogurt (Low-fat)	1 cup	14	Calories: 150, Protein: 10g, Fat: 4g, Carbs: 17g
Coconut Yogurt (Unsweetened)	1 cup	Varies	Calories: 70, Protein: 1g, Fat: 7g, Carbs: 4g

Skyr (Icelandic Yogurt)	1 cup	40	Calories: 59, Protein: 10g, Fat: 0.4g, Carbs: 4g
Butter and Butter Substitutes			
Butter (Unsalted)	1 tbsp	0	Calories: 102, Protein: 0.1g, Fat: 11.5g, Carbs: 0g
Olive Oil Spread	1 tbsp	0	Calories: 39, Protein: 0.1g, Fat: 4.4g, Carbs: 0g
Ice Cream and Frozen Desserts			
Vanilla Ice Cream (Low-fat)	1/2 cup	47	Calories: 134, Protein: 3g, Fat: 3.6g, Carbs: 23g
Frozen Yogurt (Non-fat)	1/2 cup	35	Calories: 104, Protein: 4g, Fat: 0.4g, Carbs: 22g

Almond Milk Ice Cream	1/2 cup	Varies	Calories: 200, Protein: 1g, Fat: 13g, Carbs: 20g
Cream and Cream Alternatives			
Heavy Cream	1 tbsp	0	Calories: 52, Protein: 0.4g, Fat: 5.4g, Carbs: 0.4g
Coconut Cream	1 cup	10	Calories: 330, Protein: 3g, Fat: 34g, Carbs: 6g
Cashew Cream	1 cup	Varies	Calories: 50, Protein: 2g, Fat: 4g, Carbs: 2g
Milkshakes and Smoothies			
Strawberry Milkshake	1 cup	Varies	Calories: 110, Protein: 2g, Fat: 2g, Carbs: 22g

Green Smoothie (Kale, Banana, Almond Milk)	1 cup	Varies	Calories: 50, Protein: 2g, Fat: 1g, Carbs: 11g
Condensed and Evaporated Milk			
Sweetened Condensed Milk	1 tbsp	61	Calories: 61, Protein: 0.9g, Fat: 1.7g, Carbs: 10.6g
Evaporated Milk (Low-fat)	1 cup	32	Calories: 168, Protein: 14g, Fat: 2g, Carbs: 24g
Milk Powder and Instant Milk			
Non-Fat Dry Milk	1 cup	32	Calories: 352, Protein: 32.5g, Fat: 0.6g, Carbs: 52.4g
Soy Milk Powder	1/4 cup	29	Calories: 90, Protein: 6g, Fat: 4g, Carbs: 6g

Plant-Based Creamers			
Almond Milk Creamer	1 tbsp	25	Calories: 10, Protein: 0g, Fat: 1g, Carbs: 1g
Coconut Milk Creamer	1 tbsp	20	Calories: 10, Protein: 0g, Fat: 1g, Carbs: 0g
Miscellaneous Dairy Products			
Ricotta Cheese	1/2 cup	35	Calories: 337, Protein: 14g, Fat: 27g, Carbs: 8g
Goat Cheese	1 oz	0	Calories: 103, Protein: 6g, Fat: 9g, Carbs: 0g
Yogurt Drinks			
Kefir (Plain, Low-fat)	1 cup	30	Calories: 110, Protein: 10g, Fat: 2g, Carbs: 14g
Lassi (Plain)	1 cup	Varies	Calories: 96, Protein: 3g,

			Fat: 6g, Carbs: 8g
Custards and Puddings			
Vanilla Pudding (Sugar-Free)	1/2 cup	Varies	Calories: 70, Protein: 1g, Fat: 2g, Carbs: 15g
Rice Pudding (Low-fat)	1/2 cup	87	Calories: 112, Protein: 2g, Fat: 1g, Carbs: 25g
Dairy-Based Dips			
Tzatziki (Yogurt-based)	2 tbsp	9	Calories: 39, Protein: 1g, Fat: 3g, Carbs: 2g
Spinach and Artichoke Dip	2 tbsp	Varies	Calories: 82, Protein: 2g, Fat: 7g, Carbs: 4g
Frozen Yogurt Popsicles			
Strawberry Yogurt Popsicle	1 popsicle	Varies	Calories: 27, Protein: 1g, Fat: 0g, Carbs: 7g

Chocolate Yogurt Popsicle	1 popsicle	Varies	Calories: 28, Protein: 1g, Fat: 0g, Carbs: 7g
Plant-Based Yogurt Alternatives			
Soy Yogurt (Unsweetened)	1 cup	15	Calories: 46, Protein: 4g, Fat: 2.5g, Carbs: 2.4g
Cashew Milk Yogurt (Vanilla)	1 cup	Varies	Calories: 50, Protein: 1g, Fat: 2.5g, Carbs: 5g
Cheesecake			
Greek Yogurt Cheesecake	1 slice	Varies	Calories: 290, Protein: 20g, Fat: 14g, Carbs: 22g
Milkshakes and Smoothies			
Mango Lassi Smoothie	1 cup	Varies	Calories: 150, Protein: 3g, Fat: 2g, Carbs: 32g

Strawberry Banana Smoothie	1 cup	Varies	Calories: 80, Protein: 1g, Fat: 0.5g, Carbs: 19g

These dairy and dairy alternative options provide a variety of choices for individuals managing type-2 diabetes. Always consult with a healthcare professional or a registered dietitian for personalized dietary advice.

Here's another set of 50 dairy and dairy alternative foods suitable for individuals with type-2 diabetes, presented in tabular form with columns for food type, portion sizes, approximate glycemic index (GI) values (measured on a scale of 0 to 100), and basic nutritional information per 100 grams:

Food Type	Portion Size	Low Glycemic Index	Nutritional Information (per 100g)
Milk and Dairy Substitutes			
Whole Milk	1 cup	41	Calories: 61, Protein: 3.2g, Fat: 3.3g, Carbs: 4.8g

Food Type	Portion Size	Low Glycemic Index	Nutritional Information (per 100g)
Rice Milk (Unsweetened)	1 cup	86	Calories: 47, Protein: 0.3g, Fat: 0.9g, Carbs: 9.3g
Hemp Milk	1 cup	Varies	Calories: 70, Protein: 2.7g, Fat: 5.3g, Carbs: 3.7g
Soy Milk (Unsweetened)	1 cup	22	Calories: 33, Protein: 3.3g, Fat: 1.8g, Carbs: 1.7g
Cheese and Cheese Alternatives			
Mozzarella Cheese (Part-skim)	1 oz	0	Calories: 72, Protein: 7.4g, Fat: 4.5g, Carbs: 0.6g
Vegan Cheddar Cheese	1 slice	Varies	Calories: 80, Protein: 2g, Fat: 7g, Carbs: 1g

Food Type	Portion Size	Low Glycemic Index	Nutritional Information (per 100g)
Swiss Cheese	1 oz	0	Calories: 98, Protein: 7g, Fat: 7.9g, Carbs: 2.2g
Cashew Cheese	1 oz	Varies	Calories: 74, Protein: 2g, Fat: 5.9g, Carbs: 3.5g
Yogurt and Yogurt Alternatives			
Regular Yogurt (Full-fat)	1 cup	14	Calories: 149, Protein: 3.5g, Fat: 8g, Carbs: 14g
Almond Milk Yogurt (Vanilla)	1 cup	Varies	Calories: 50, Protein: 1g, Fat: 2.5g, Carbs: 5g
Low-Fat Greek Yogurt	1 cup	11	Calories: 59, Protein: 10g, Fat: 0.4g, Carbs: 3.6g

Food Type	Portion Size	Low Glycemic Index	Nutritional Information (per 100g)
Coconut Milk Yogurt (Unsweetened)	1 cup	Varies	Calories: 70, Protein: 1g, Fat: 7g, Carbs: 4g
Butter and Butter Substitutes			
Ghee	1 tbsp	0	Calories: 112, Protein: 0g, Fat: 12g, Carbs: 0g
Margarine (Soft, Unsaturated)	1 tbsp	0	Calories: 102, Protein: 0.1g, Fat: 11.5g, Carbs: 0.1g
Ice Cream and Frozen Desserts			
Chocolate Ice Cream (Low-fat)	1/2 cup	Varies	Calories: 143, Protein: 3.2g, Fat: 2.9g, Carbs: 28.9g
Sorbet (Various Flavors)	1/2 cup	Varies	Calories: 95, Protein: 0.5g,

Food Type	Portion Size	Low Glycemic Index	Nutritional Information (per 100g)
			Fat: 0.3g, Carbs: 25g
Coconut Milk Ice Cream (Vanilla)	1/2 cup	Varies	Calories: 200, Protein: 1g, Fat: 13g, Carbs: 20g
Cream and Cream Alternatives			
Half-and-Half Cream	1 tbsp	0	Calories: 20, Protein: 0.6g, Fat: 1.7g, Carbs: 0.6g
Soy Cream	1 tbsp	Varies	Calories: 43, Protein: 0.3g, Fat: 4.4g, Carbs: 1g
Milkshakes and Smoothies			
Chocolate Milkshake (Low-fat)	1 cup	Varies	Calories: 150, Protein: 6g, Fat: 2g, Carbs: 27g

Food Type	Portion Size	Low Glycemic Index	Nutritional Information (per 100g)
Blueberry Smoothie (Yogurt-based)	1 cup	Varies	Calories: 70, Protein: 1g, Fat: 0.5g, Carbs: 18g
Condensed and Evaporated Milk			
Sweetened Condensed Milk	1 tbsp	61	Calories: 61, Protein: 0.9g, Fat: 1.7g, Carbs: 10.6g
Evaporated Milk (Whole)	1 cup	32	Calories: 338, Protein: 17g, Fat: 20g, Carbs: 27g
Milk Powder and Instant Milk			
Skimmed Milk Powder	1 cup	32	Calories: 362, Protein: 34g, Fat: 1g, Carbs: 52g
Oat Milk Powder	1/4 cup	Varies	Calories: 84, Protein: 1.6g,

Food Type	Portion Size	Low Glycemic Index	Nutritional Information (per 100g)
			Fat: 1.3g, Carbs: 16g
Plant-Based Creamers			
Hazelnut Milk Creamer	1 tbsp	0	Calories: 20, Protein: 0g, Fat: 2g, Carbs: 0g
Oat Milk Creamer	1 tbsp	Varies	Calories: 13, Protein: 0.2g, Fat: 1.2g, Carbs: 0.4g
Miscellaneous Dairy Products			
Quark Cheese	1 cup	15	Calories: 72, Protein: 12g, Fat: 0.5g, Carbs: 3.9g
Blue Cheese	1 oz	0	Calories: 100, Protein: 6g, Fat: 8g, Carbs: 0.7g
Yogurt Drinks			

Food Type	Portion Size	Low Glycemic Index	Nutritional Information (per 100g)
Drinkable Yogurt (Strawberry)	1 bottle	Varies	Calories: 150, Protein: 6g, Fat: 2.5g, Carbs: 28g
Ayran (Yogurt Drink)	1 cup	Varies	Calories: 52, Protein: 3g, Fat: 2.1g, Carbs: 4.8g
Custards and Puddings			
Chocolate Pudding (Sugar-Free)	1/2 cup	Varies	Calories: 90, Protein: 2g, Fat: 0.5g, Carbs: 21g
Tapioca Pudding (Low-fat)	1/2 cup	58	Calories: 102, Protein: 2.4g, Fat: 0.2g, Carbs: 23g
Dairy-Based Dips			
Roquefort Dressing	2 tbsp	0	Calories: 149, Protein: 1.5g,

Food Type	Portion Size	Low Glycemic Index	Nutritional Information (per 100g)
			Fat: 16g, Carbs: 1.5g
Yogurt and Dill Dip	2 tbsp	0	Calories: 46, Protein: 1.6g, Fat: 4.2g, Carbs: 1.2g
Frozen Yogurt Popsicles			
Peach Yogurt Popsicle	1 popsicle	Varies	Calories: 27, Protein: 1g, Fat: 0g, Carbs: 7g
Raspberry Yogurt Popsicle	1 popsicle	Varies	Calories: 28, Protein: 1g, Fat: 0g, Carbs: 7g
Plant-Based Yogurt Alternatives			
Almond Milk Yogurt (Unsweetened)	1 cup	Varies	Calories: 13, Protein: 0.5g, Fat: 0.8g, Carbs: 1.3g

Food Type	Portion Size	Low Glycemic Index	Nutritional Information (per 100g)
Coconut Milk Yogurt (Vanilla)	1 cup	Varies	Calories: 120, Protein: 1g, Fat: 2g, Carbs: 23g
Cheesecake			
Low-Fat Blueberry Cheesecake	1 slice	Varies	Calories: 240, Protein: 9g, Fat: 5g, Carbs: 40g
Milkshakes and Smoothies			
Banana Peanut Butter Smoothie	1 cup	Varies	Calories: 160, Protein: 5g, Fat: 8g, Carbs: 18g
Green Tea Milkshake	1 cup	Varies	Calories: 120, Protein: 3g, Fat: 2g, Carbs: 26g

These additional dairy and dairy alternative options offer a diverse range for individuals managing type-2 diabetes. Always consult with a healthcare professional or a registered dietitian for personalized dietary advice.

HERBS AND SPICES

Here's a table featuring 50 herbs and spicy foods suitable for individuals with type-2 diabetes. The table includes information on food type, portion sizes, approximate glycemic index (GI) values (measured on a scale of 0 to 100), and basic nutritional information per 100 grams:

Food Type	Portion Size	Low Glycemic Index	Nutritional Information (per 100g)
Herbs and Spices			
Basil	1 tbsp	0	Calories: 23, Protein: 3.2g, Fat: 0.6g, Carbs: 2.7g
Cilantro	1 tbsp	0	Calories: 23, Protein: 2.1g, Fat: 0.5g, Carbs: 3.7g
Thyme	1 tsp	0	Calories: 101, Protein: 5.6g, Fat: 1.7g, Carbs: 24.4g
Rosemary	1 tsp	0	Calories: 131, Protein: 3.3g, Fat: 5.9g, Carbs: 20.7g

Food Type	Portion Size	Low Glycemic Index	Nutritional Information (per 100g)
Chilies and Peppers			
Cayenne Pepper	1 tsp	Varies	Calories: 17, Protein: 0.9g, Fat: 0.6g, Carbs: 3.7g
Jalapeno Pepper	1 pepper	Varies	Calories: 29, Protein: 1.4g, Fat: 0.4g, Carbs: 6g
Bell Pepper (Green)	1 medium	10	Calories: 20, Protein: 0.9g, Fat: 0.2g, Carbs: 4.6g
Bell Pepper (Red)	1 medium	10	Calories: 31, Protein: 1.3g, Fat: 0.3g, Carbs: 6.3g
Garlic and Onions			
Garlic	1 clove	0	Calories: 149, Protein: 6.4g, Fat: 0.5g, Carbs: 33g
Onion (Yellow)	1 medium	10	Calories: 44, Protein: 1.2g, Fat: 0.1g, Carbs: 10.1g

Food Type	Portion Size	Low Glycemic Index	Nutritional Information (per 100g)
Shallots	1 medium	10	Calories: 72, Protein: 2.5g, Fat: 0.1g, Carbs: 17.1g
Leeks	1 cup	10	Calories: 61, Protein: 1.5g, Fat: 0.3g, Carbs: 14.2g
Cumin and Coriander			
Ground Cumin	1 tsp	0	Calories: 16, Protein: 0.9g, Fat: 1g, Carbs: 2.3g
Ground Coriander	1 tsp	0	Calories: 23, Protein: 0.6g, Fat: 0.5g, Carbs: 4.4g
Turmeric and Ginger			
Turmeric	1 tsp	Varies	Calories: 29, Protein: 0.9g, Fat: 0.3g, Carbs: 6.3g

Food Type	Portion Size	Low Glycemic Index	Nutritional Information (per 100g)
Fresh Ginger	1 tbsp	Varies	Calories: 18, Protein: 0.6g, Fat: 0.2g, Carbs: 4g
Oregano and Sage			
Dried Oregano	1 tsp	0	Calories: 265, Protein: 9g, Fat: 4.3g, Carbs: 68.9g
Fresh Sage	1 tbsp	0	Calories: 43, Protein: 1.6g, Fat: 0.6g, Carbs: 8.1g
Cinnamon and Nutmeg			
Ground Cinnamon	1 tsp	Varies	Calories: 247, Protein: 4g, Fat: 1.2g, Carbs: 80.6g
Ground Nutmeg	1 tsp	Varies	Calories: 525, Protein: 5.8g, Fat: 36.3g, Carbs: 49.2g

Food Type	Portion Size	Low Glycemic Index	Nutritional Information (per 100g)
Basil Pesto and Cilantro Pesto			
Basil Pesto	1 tbsp	0	Calories: 150, Protein: 2g, Fat: 15g, Carbs: 2g
Cilantro Pesto	1 tbsp	0	Calories: 71, Protein: 1g, Fat: 7g, Carbs: 2g
Paprika and Chili Powder			
Sweet Paprika	1 tsp	0	Calories: 20, Protein: 1g, Fat: 0.9g, Carbs: 4.2g
Chili Powder	1 tsp	Varies	Calories: 24, Protein: 1.5g, Fat: 1.3g, Carbs: 4.8g
Cayenne and Black Pepper			
Cayenne Pepper	1 tsp	Varies	Calories: 17, Protein: 0.9g, Fat: 0.6g, Carbs: 3.7g

Food Type	Portion Size	Low Glycemic Index	Nutritional Information (per 100g)
Black Pepper	1 tsp	Varies	Calories: 5, Protein: 0.1g, Fat: 0.1g, Carbs: 1.3g
Parsley and Dill			
Fresh Parsley	1 tbsp	0	Calories: 1, Protein: 0.1g, Fat: 0g, Carbs: 0.2g
Fresh Dill	1 tbsp	0	Calories: 6, Protein: 0.5g, Fat: 0.2g, Carbs: 1g
Paprika and Red Pepper Flakes			
Smoked Paprika	1 tsp	Varies	Calories: 19, Protein: 0.9g, Fat: 0.9g, Carbs: 3.7g
Red Pepper Flakes	1 tsp	Varies	Calories: 29, Protein: 1.3g, Fat: 1.3g, Carbs: 5.9g
Curry Powder and Bay Leaves			

Food Type	Portion Size	Low Glycemic Index	Nutritional Information (per 100g)
Curry Powder	1 tsp	Varies	Calories: 325, Protein: 9.2g, Fat: 14.3g, Carbs: 64.8g
Bay Leaves	1 leaf	0	Calories: 313, Protein: 7.6g, Fat: 8.4g, Carbs: 75.8g
Garlic Powder and Onion Powder			
Garlic Powder	1 tsp	Varies	Calories: 331, Protein: 16.3g, Fat: 0.5g, Carbs: 72.7g
Onion Powder	1 tsp	Varies	Calories: 342, Protein: 10.4g, Fat: 1.2g, Carbs: 74.9g
Cajun Seasoning and Italian Seasoning			

Food Type	Portion Size	Low Glycemic Index	Nutritional Information (per 100g)
Cajun Seasoning	1 tsp	Varies	Calories: 8, Protein: 0.3g, Fat: 0.4g, Carbs: 1.6g
Italian Seasoning	1 tsp	Varies	Calories: 255, Protein: 11.9g, Fat: 4.3g, Carbs: 64.1g

Including these herbs and spices in your diet can add flavor without significantly impacting blood sugar levels. Always consult with a healthcare professional or a registered dietitian for personalized dietary advice.

Here's another set of 50 herbs and spicy foods suitable for individuals with type-2 diabetes, presented in tabular form with columns for food type, portion sizes, approximate glycemic index (GI) values (measured on a scale of 0 to 100), and basic nutritional information per 100 grams:

Food Type	Portion Size	Low Glycemic Index	Nutritional Information (per 100g)
Herbs and Spices			
Mint	1 tbsp	0	Calories: 70, Protein: 3.3g, Fat: 0.9g, Carbs: 14.9g
Chives	1 tbsp	0	Calories: 30, Protein: 1.9g, Fat: 0.7g, Carbs: 4.4g
Tarragon	1 tbsp	0	Calories: 295, Protein: 22.8g, Fat: 7.4g, Carbs: 50.2g
Dill	1 tbsp	0	Calories: 43, Protein: 2.1g, Fat: 0.6g, Carbs: 7.9g
Cayenne and Chili Peppers			
Chili Pepper Flakes	1 tsp	Varies	Calories: 40, Protein: 2g, Fat: 2g, Carbs: 8g

Anaheim Pepper	1 medium	Varies	Calories: 18, Protein: 1g, Fat: 0g, Carbs: 4g
Habanero Pepper	1 pepper	Varies	Calories: 30, Protein: 1.3g, Fat: 0.6g, Carbs: 6.7g
Shishito Pepper	1 oz	Varies	Calories: 15, Protein: 1g, Fat: 0g, Carbs: 3g
Garlic and Onions			
Roasted Garlic	1 clove	0	Calories: 149, Protein: 6.4g, Fat: 0.5g, Carbs: 33g
Red Onion	1 medium	10	Calories: 40, Protein: 1.1g, Fat: 0.1g, Carbs: 9.3g
Green Onion	1 stalk	10	Calories: 32, Protein: 1.6g, Fat: 0.2g, Carbs: 7.3g
Pearl Onion	1 cup	10	Calories: 28, Protein: 1.2g,

			Fat: 0.1g, Carbs: 6.7g
Coriander and Fennel			
Fresh Coriander	1 tbsp	0	Calories: 23, Protein: 2.1g, Fat: 0.5g, Carbs: 3.7g
Fennel Seeds	1 tsp	0	Calories: 345, Protein: 15.8g, Fat: 14.9g, Carbs: 52.3g
Ground Coriander	1 tsp	0	Calories: 23, Protein: 0.6g, Fat: 0.5g, Carbs: 4.4g
Ginger and Turmeric			
Ground Ginger	1 tsp	Varies	Calories: 80, Protein: 1.8g, Fat: 0.8g, Carbs: 18g
Fresh Turmeric	1 inch piece	Varies	Calories: 65, Protein: 3.1g, Fat: 0.7g, Carbs: 14.1g
Ground Turmeric	1 tsp	Varies	Calories: 312, Protein: 9.7g,

			Fat: 3.2g, Carbs: 67.1g
Parsley and Sage			
Flat-leaf Parsley	1 tbsp	0	Calories: 36, Protein: 2.2g, Fat: 0.8g, Carbs: 6.3g
Sage	1 tbsp	0	Calories: 315, Protein: 10.6g, Fat: 1.7g, Carbs: 64.1g
Dried Sage	1 tsp	0	Calories: 315, Protein: 10.6g, Fat: 1.7g, Carbs: 64.1g
Cinnamon and Nutmeg			
Cinnamon	1 tsp	Varies	Calories: 247, Protein: 4g, Fat: 1.2g, Carbs: 80.6g
Nutmeg	1 tsp	Varies	Calories: 525, Protein: 5.8g, Fat: 36.3g, Carbs: 49.2g

Basil Pesto and Cilantro Pesto			
Basil Pesto	1 tbsp	0	Calories: 150, Protein: 2g, Fat: 15g, Carbs: 2g
Cilantro Pesto	1 tbsp	0	Calories: 71, Protein: 1g, Fat: 7g, Carbs: 2g
Paprika and Chili Powder			
Smoked Paprika	1 tsp	Varies	Calories: 19, Protein: 0.9g, Fat: 0.9g, Carbs: 3.7g
Chipotle Chili Powder	1 tsp	Varies	Calories: 16, Protein: 1g, Fat: 0.9g, Carbs: 3.1g
Cumin and Cardamom			
Ground Cumin	1 tsp	0	Calories: 16, Protein: 0.9g, Fat: 1g, Carbs: 2.3g

Ground Cardamom	1 tsp	0	Calories: 311, Protein: 10.8g, Fat: 6.7g, Carbs: 68.5g
Rosemary and Oregano			
Fresh Rosemary	1 tbsp	0	Calories: 131, Protein: 3.3g, Fat: 5.9g, Carbs: 20.7g
Dried Oregano	1 tsp	0	Calories: 265, Protein: 9g, Fat: 4.3g, Carbs: 68.9g
Paprika and Red Pepper Flakes			
Sweet Paprika	1 tsp	0	Calories: 20, Protein: 1g, Fat: 0.9g, Carbs: 4.2g
Red Pepper Flakes	1 tsp	Varies	Calories: 29, Protein: 1.3g, Fat: 1.3g, Carbs: 5.9g
Curry Powder and Bay Leaves			

Yellow Curry Powder	1 tsp	Varies	Calories: 325, Protein: 9.2g, Fat: 14.3g, Carbs: 64.8g
Bay Leaves	1 leaf	0	Calories: 313, Protein: 7.6g, Fat: 8.4g, Carbs: 75.8g
Garlic Powder and Onion Powder			
Granulated Garlic	1 tsp	Varies	Calories: 331, Protein: 16.3g, Fat: 0.5g, Carbs: 72.7g
Onion Powder	1 tsp	Varies	Calories: 342, Protein: 10.4g, Fat: 1.2g, Carbs: 74.9g
Cajun Seasoning and Italian Seasoning			
Cajun Seasoning	1 tsp	Varies	Calories: 8, Protein: 0.3g, Fat: 0.4g, Carbs: 1.6g

Italian Seasoning	1 tsp	Varies	Calories: 255, Protein: 11.9g, Fat: 4.3g, Carbs: 64.1g

Including these additional herbs and spices in your diet can enhance the flavor of your meals without significantly impacting blood sugar levels. Always consult with a healthcare professional or a registered dietitian for personalized dietary advice.

CHAPTER 6

MEAL PLANNING AND RECIPES

6.1 Sample Meal Plans

Creating well-balanced and nutritious meal plans is crucial for individuals managing Type-2 Diabetes. A thoughtful approach to meal planning can help regulate blood sugar levels, manage weight, and promote overall health. Here are some sample meal plans designed with a focus on variety, portion control, and nutritional balance.

Sample Meal Plan 1: Mediterranean Delight

Breakfast:

- Greek Yogurt Parfait with Fresh Berries and a sprinkle of Chia Seeds
- Whole-grain Toast with Avocado

Lunch:

- Grilled Chicken Salad with a variety of colorful vegetables (tomatoes, cucumbers, bell peppers)
- Quinoa and Chickpea Mediterranean Bowl

Dinner:

- Baked Salmon with Lemon and Dill
- Roasted Sweet Potatoes

- Steamed Broccoli with Garlic

Snacks:

- Almonds and Walnuts Mix
- Fresh Fruit Salad

Sample Meal Plan 2: Plant-Powered Day

Breakfast:

- Oatmeal topped with Sliced Banana and a drizzle of Honey
- Green Smoothie with Spinach, Banana, and Almond Milk

Lunch:

- Lentil and Vegetable Soup
- Whole-grain Wrap with Hummus, Spinach, and Roasted Vegetables

Dinner:

- Quinoa-Stuffed Bell Peppers with Black Beans and Corn
- Grilled Zucchini and Eggplant

Snacks:

- Celery Sticks with Peanut Butter
- Cherry Tomatoes with Feta Cheese

Sample Meal Plan 3: Balanced Plate

Breakfast:

- Scrambled Eggs with Spinach and Tomatoes
- Whole-grain English Muffin

Lunch:

- Turkey and Avocado Wrap with Whole-grain Tortilla
- Mixed Greens Salad with Olive Oil and Balsamic Vinegar Dressing

Dinner:

- Baked Chicken Breast with Rosemary
- Quinoa Pilaf with Mixed Vegetables
- Steamed Asparagus

Snacks:

- Cottage Cheese with Pineapple
- Handful of Mixed Berries

These sample meal plans emphasize the importance of incorporating a variety of nutrient-dense foods, including lean proteins, whole grains, healthy fats, and plenty of colorful vegetables. It's essential to monitor portion sizes and be mindful of carbohydrate intake to maintain stable blood sugar levels.

6.2 Recipe Ideas for Balanced Meals

Creating delicious and diabetes-friendly meals doesn't have to be complicated. Here are some recipe ideas that focus on flavor, nutrition, and balance:

Recipe 1: Grilled Salmon with Lemon-Dill Sauce

Ingredients:

- 4 salmon fillets
- 2 tablespoons olive oil
- Juice of 1 lemon
- 1 tablespoon chopped fresh dill
- Salt and pepper to taste

Instructions:

1. Preheat the grill to medium-high heat.
2. Rub salmon fillets with olive oil and season with salt and pepper.
3. Grill salmon for 4-5 minutes per side or until cooked through.
4. In a small bowl, mix lemon juice and chopped dill to create the sauce.
5. Drizzle the lemon-dill sauce over grilled salmon before serving.

Recipe 2: Quinoa and Chickpea Mediterranean Bowl

Ingredients:

- 1 cup cooked quinoa
- 1 can chickpeas, drained and rinsed
- Cherry tomatoes, halved
- Cucumber, diced
- Kalamata olives, sliced
- Feta cheese, crumbled
- Olive oil and balsamic vinegar for dressing

Instructions:

1. In a bowl, combine cooked quinoa, chickpeas, cherry tomatoes, cucumber, olives, and feta cheese.
2. Drizzle olive oil and balsamic vinegar over the ingredients and toss gently.
3. Serve the Mediterranean bowl chilled.

Recipe 3: Lentil and Vegetable Soup

Ingredients:

- 1 cup dry green or brown lentils, rinsed
- 1 onion, diced
- 2 carrots, sliced
- 2 celery stalks, chopped

- 3 cloves garlic, minced
- 1 can diced tomatoes
- 6 cups vegetable broth
- 1 teaspoon cumin
- 1 teaspoon paprika
- Salt and pepper to taste
- Fresh parsley for garnish

Instructions:

1. In a large pot, sauté onions, carrots, celery, and garlic until softened.
2. Add lentils, diced tomatoes, vegetable broth, cumin, paprika, salt, and pepper.
3. Bring to a boil, then reduce heat and simmer for 25-30 minutes or until lentils are tender.
4. Garnish with fresh parsley before serving.

6.3 Cooking Tips for Diabetes-Friendly Meals

Cooking for diabetes involves making mindful choices to manage blood sugar levels while ensuring that meals remain enjoyable. Here are some cooking tips to assist in preparing diabetes-friendly meals:

Tip 1: Choose Whole, Unprocessed Foods

Opt for whole grains, fresh fruits, vegetables, lean proteins, and healthy fats. Avoid highly processed and refined foods, as they often contain added sugars and can cause rapid spikes in blood sugar.

Tip 2: Embrace Lean Proteins

Include lean protein sources like poultry, fish, tofu, beans, and legumes in your meals. Protein helps stabilize blood sugar levels and promotes a feeling of fullness.

Tip 3: Prioritize Fiber

Fiber-rich foods, such as whole grains, legumes, and vegetables, play a crucial role in managing blood sugar. They slow down the absorption of glucose and contribute to overall digestive health.

Tip 4: Be Mindful of Portion Sizes

Controlling portion sizes is key to managing calorie intake and blood sugar levels. Use smaller plates and be aware of recommended serving sizes for different food groups.

Tip 5: Healthy Cooking Methods

Opt for cooking methods like grilling, baking, steaming, and sautéing instead of frying. These methods retain the nutritional value of foods without adding excessive fats.

Tip 6: Monitor Carbohydrate Intake

While carbohydrates are an essential part of a balanced diet, it's important to monitor and distribute them evenly throughout the day. This helps prevent sharp increases in blood sugar levels.

Tip 7: Experiment with Herbs and Spices

Enhance the flavor of your meals without relying on excessive salt or sugar. Experiment with a variety of herbs and spices to add depth and complexity to your dishes.

Tip 8: Stay Hydrated

Drinking enough water is essential for overall health and can aid in managing blood sugar levels. Aim for at least eight glasses of water per day.

Tip 9: Plan and Prep Ahead

Planning meals in advance and preparing ingredients ahead of time can help you make healthier choices and avoid the temptation of convenient but less nutritious options.

Tip 10: Regularly Monitor Blood Sugar Levels

Keep track of your blood sugar levels regularly, especially after meals, to understand how different foods affect your body. This information can guide future meal choices.

By incorporating these sample meal plans, recipes, and cooking tips into your routine, you can enjoy a diverse and satisfying diet while effectively managing Type-2 Diabetes. Remember, consulting with a healthcare professional or a registered dietitian for personalized advice is always recommended.

Printed in Great Britain
by Amazon